EMBRACING THE LIZARD

A GUIDE TO MEDITATION TOOLS AND TECHNIQUES

SEEMA VIKRAM SURANA

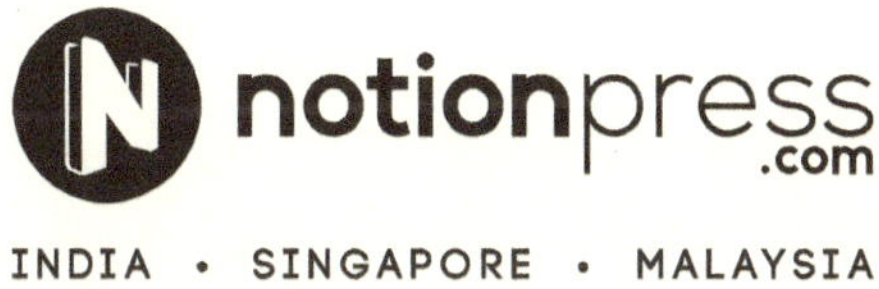

INDIA • SINGAPORE • MALAYSIA

ISBN
Paperback: 979-8-89632-455-3
Hardcase: 979-8-89699-417-6

TO

Vikram, whose memory is etched in my heart like the sunset's warmth on my skin.

Vikram, whose memory lives on in every breath of mine.

Your impact on my life has been profound, and I honour your memory by dedicating **my book EMBRACING THE LIZARD** *to you.*

Your legacy and goodwill continue to guide me, illuminating my path and inspiring me to embrace life's challenges with courage and resilience.

With love and gratitude, always.

CONTENTS

Foreword 7

Acknowledgement 9

Overview of the Book 11

Introduction 13

Chapter 1: The Lizard's Secret 17

Chapter 2: The Concept of Peaceful Presence and Meditation 20

Chapter 3: Nadis, Chakras, and Mudras 24

Chapter 4: External Tools: Aids for Enhancing Meditation 30

Chapter 5: Internal Tools Navigating Peaceful Presence 41

- N - Now 44
- A - Awareness 47
- V - For Visualisation 50
- I - Intuition 53
- G - Gratitude 55

A - Affirmation and Mantras 58

T - Transformation 70

I - Integrating 72

N - Nourishment 76

G - Grounding 84

Chapter 6: Practices 87

Conclusion *99*

FOREWORD

If you've ever felt that peace and calmness are more than just fleeting moments, *Embracing The Lizard* from the author Seema Surana is your essential guide. This playful yet profound book explores the art of meditation, mindfulness, and self-discovery, offering a refreshing perspective on how to integrate tranquillity into everyday life.

As a Mind Performance coach and the author of the bestseller *Unleash the Power of Reading,* I understand the importance of mental clarity and emotional balance in achieving a fulfilling and purposeful life. The journey toward inner peace can feel elusive, but it also holds the potential for profound transformation. This book provides practical tools and actionable insights to help you navigate this journey with ease and confidence.

What makes *Embracing The Lizard* truly unique is its ability to blend humour, practical wisdom, and scientifically-backed techniques. Through relatable metaphors and guided exercises, the book demonstrates how mindfulness and meditation can awaken your senses, overcome common obstacles, and cultivate a deep sense of serenity. It offers strategies not just to quiet the mind but to embrace life with a sense of presence and purpose.

This book challenges us to see meditation as more than a practice – it's a way of being, a pathway to living fully in the present moment. It inspires readers to pause, breathe, and embrace the calmness already within them, unlocking a deeper connection to their inner selves.

Whether you are new to meditation, a seasoned practitioner, or someone seeking balance in a chaotic world, *Embracing The Lizard* is a must-read. It will empower you to bask in the sunlight of mindfulness and thrive in the warmth of your own inner peace.

Best wishes,

Manjunath MS
MIND PERFORMANCE COACH

(Dr. Manjunath M.S.)

Mind Performance Coach and
Author of *Unleash the Power of Reading*

ACKNOWLEDGEMENT

The amazing dedication of spiritual leaders like Sadguru, Jain Acharya Tulsiji, Acharya Mahapragyaji, and Acharya Mahashramanji for sharing their spiritual wisdom is truly inspiring. "Their teachings and writings lit a burning desire within Vikram and me, and because of them, I could experience positive changes in myself and am still experiencing changes in self-growth.

I extend my heartfelt gratitude to the following individuals who played a vital role in bringing this book to life.

Firstly, I thank Notion Press, my publisher, for believing in this project and expertly guiding it to publication.

Next, I appreciate my exceptional editor, whose skill and dedication refined my work.

Dr Manjunath, M.S. speed reading, memory, and mind performance coach deserves special thanks for his invaluable guidance.

On a personal note, I thank my children, Ayush, Shweta, and Ritika, for their unwavering support and encouragement. Their technical expertise and enthusiasm helped me navigate challenges.

To my loving family and friends - Vinod, Shobha, Vinay, Sonal, Sudha, Abhishek, Hema, Kailash, Prem, and Naresh - thank you for your unconditional love and support.

Lastly, I honour Vikram's parents Vijaya Devi Surana and Prem Chandji Surana, and my parents Chanda Devi Begani, and Jyoti Kumarji Begani—whose love and inspiration have shaped my life's journey. I love you all. You are my greatest friends. Your contributions, big or small, have made this book a reality. I cherish your presence in my life.

Special thanks to Vikram, with whom I spent 25 years of my life. This book is a testament to your collective support and inspiration.

With sincere gratitude, I honour the beautiful souls who've touched my life, who have had a profound impact on me, and who have been offering support, encouragement, and insight. Your presence has been a blessing, helping me grow, learn, and shine.

OVERVIEW OF THE BOOK

Finding peace can feel as vague as a lizard in a sunbeam – quick and slippery. But what if, instead of chasing after tranquillity, you could learn to embrace it with the skill and charm of your inner lizard? Picture yourself basking in the warmth of calmness, just like that little reptile soaking up the sun, completely unbothered by the chaos around it.

Embracing The Lizard is a playful yet profound guide to discovering meditation tools and techniques to help you open to inner peace, mindfulness, and self-discovery. With a touch of humour and plenty of practical wisdom, this book shows you that serenity isn't just a far-off dream—it's something you can find right under your nose, or perhaps right on your favourite sunlit rock.

Within these pages, you'll discover:

- **Techniques of meditation that have been proven to quiet the mind by waking up your senses and tapping your inner wisdom too.**
- **How some practical tools and exercises can cultivate concentration, mindfulness, and emotional balance.**
- **Guided meditation which will help you to overcome common obstacles and challenges while meditating.**

- **Benefits of meditation and inner peace on our physical appearance as well as our mental and emotional well-being, which are scientifically proven.**

INTRODUCTION

The story behind this book

In 2015, our family was shaken to its core when Vikram, my husband, was diagnosed with blood cancer, filling us with fear and anxiety. It felt like a heavy blanket suffocating us. During treatment, a small lizard appeared, becoming an unlikely friend. Vikram, who once feared reptiles, now shared his space with it. The lizard's presence made us feel uneasy, yet curious. Each night, its quiet presence challenged our fears. One night, Vikram screamed after a powerful dream.

In his dream, a lizard appeared before him, saying, "Don't judge me by my appearance. See beyond my looks and admire my strengths." The lizard then revealed its remarkable qualities: adaptability, quiet courage, and unwavering presence. Its words were like gold, filled with wisdom and insight.

After learning about the dream, we were left pondering how to embark on our new journey. We eagerly awaited nightfall, hoping to glimpse the lizard and gain some insight. As we gazed at the lizard, its presence struck us. We saw how it adapted, stayed strong, and kept showing up. This tiny creature inspired us to face our challenges with courage and determination. It became a symbol of our resilience and a reminder that we too can overcome anything.

We were deeply moved, especially Vikram, and his heart transformed. The lizard, as a creature to fear, was now a symbol of resilience. From that moment on, we looked at the world with new eyes, seeking the hidden strengths in all beings.

A deep silence fell between us as we searched for life's purpose. One day, Vikram expressed his desire to write a book about his journey, inspiring fellow patients and guiding others on their path to self-discovery.

I found my life's purpose in supporting Vikram's aspiration to write a book. But a big question loomed: how could we write a book about meditation and growth without experience?

This thought brought me back to my experience of teaching children in Gyan Shala, founded by Acharya Tulsi.

Acharya Tulsi, a visionary spiritual leader, noticed a significant gap in society's approach to emotional, mental, and spiritual well-being. He saw that education focused mainly on academic achievement, overlooking the holistic growth of children. He believed deeply in the importance of introducing spiritual values early in life, helping children grow into enlightened individuals. To bridge this gap, he launched the Gyan Shala movement in the 1960s, establishing centres dedicated to spiritual education. These centres aimed to nurture not just intellect but also emotional intelligence, values, and moral principles. His successor, Acharya Mahapragya, took this vision further by introducing engaging ways for children to explore their spiritual and emotional potential. Inspired by their teachings, in 1993 I decided to train myself as a teacher under their guidance and joined Gyan Shala. At that time, I realised how important it is to plant strong roots in children by instilling spiritual values and emotional intelligence from a young age.

I once worked with a student who had difficulty managing anger. Through the techniques taught at Gyan Shala, this student transformed into a compassionate and confident individual.

My 20 years of teaching spiritual values and emotional intelligence at Gyan Shala not only allowed me to guide children toward calmness but also helped me discover my inner peace and work harmoniously with Vikram. This sense of tranquillity became our anchor through life's challenges, helping us release past burdens and remain present. Like a lizard effortlessly adapting to its surroundings, we learned to navigate difficulties with grace, rising above them with resilience.

Life's journey transformed us, strengthening our bond and inner selves. Vikram learned to face challenges with courage and peace. But life had another chapter in store. Vikram's voyage on earth came full circle, and he embarked on a new journey, leaving me to continue ours alone. In the silence, I realised that **life's preciousness is measured in moments, not years. Every breath is a gift, every memory a treasure**. I feel Vikram's presence in every wave, breeze, and sunset. His legacy guides me, illuminating my path. I navigate life's challenges with a calmer heart, grateful for our time together.

Inspired by the lizard's resilience, adaptability, and quiet strength, Vikram's unfulfilled dream of writing a book, along with my own transformation, motivated me to create this guide to help others find serenity. This book captures the essence of spiritual wisdom from India's esteemed gurus and makes it accessible and practical for everyday life. By taking small, mindful steps, readers can cultivate inner peace and tranquillity.

Each chapter offers a clear path to achieving a peaceful presence. I invite you to join me on this journey, embracing the transformative power of these timeless principles. Like the lizard, which not only adapts but thrives by shedding its old skin, we too can shed our past burdens and emerge renewed, ready to embrace a life of inner peace.

CHAPTER 1

THE LIZARD'S SECRET

Discovering Meditation in Nature's Stillness

Have you ever watched a lizard basking in the sun, sitting perfectly still for long periods of time?

Seeing how calm and focused it is, fully present in the moment without getting distracted, is fascinating.

This state of being is similar to what we try to reach in meditation—where the mind and body are calm, fully aware, and focused on the present moment.

Imagine your mind as a busy highway, with over 60,000 thoughts zooming by every day. That's a lot of traffic! These thoughts pile up, burying the calm, quiet part of your mind under a heap of mental clutter. But here's the good news: meditation is like a peaceful detour, guiding you back to that hidden calm.

Think of your mind as an empty bowl. You can fill it with whatever you want—peace, clarity, or even that song stuck in your head. The choice is yours. Now, lizards, those chilled-out reptiles, have the right idea—they only move when necessary, saving their energy. Meditation works the same way. It helps us stop wasting mental energy on unnecessary clutter, so we can focus on what matters. The result? A clear, focused mind that's as cool as a lizard on a sunny rock.

Steve Jobs once emphasised the power of meditation, saying, "If you just sit and observe, you will see how restless your mind is. If you try to calm it, it only makes it worse, but over time it does calm, and when it does, there's room to hear more subtle things—that's when your intuition starts to blossom and you start to see things more clearly and be in the present more." With consistent meditation, we become more in tune with the details of our inner world, which helps us stay present and respond thoughtfully to whatever life throws our way.

Picture yourself as a surfer learning to ride the waves. Initially, the ocean seems daunting, and finding your balance is tough. But with time and practice, you start to sync with the rhythm of the waves, staying calm and adjusting as needed until you can ride with confidence. Meditation teaches us something similar—we observe our thoughts without getting lost in them, developing a calm, focused mind that helps us navigate life's challenges more smoothly.

Now, think of a lizard, small but resilient, surviving even the toughest weather. Despite its size, it remains steady and adaptable, much like meditation teaching us to ride the waves of life with grace. By practising mindfulness and staying in the moment, we develop the ability to handle life's challenges calmly and confidently. Just as a surfer learns to balance on the waves, we can learn to maintain our inner peace, regardless of what comes our way.

Here are simplified explanations of meditation:

1. General Explanation

Meditation is a mental practice that focuses on relaxation and concentration. It usually occurs in a quiet setting where you sit or lie comfortably, often with your eyes closed. The purpose is to train your mind to focus better, helping you gain more control over your thoughts and improve your overall mental well-being.

2. **Psychological Explanation**

   Meditation is a technique where you focus on things like your breath, a specific thought, or an object to achieve better awareness and concentration. This practice is meant to reduce stress, improve emotional control, and boost cognitive function.

3. **Spiritual Explanation**

   Meditation is a spiritual practice that seeks to bring you inner peace, a sense of connection with a higher power, or a deeper connection to the universe. It uses techniques that calm your mind, open your heart, and help you find a greater sense of purpose and spiritual understanding.

4. **Neuroscientific Explanation**

   Meditation is a mental exercise that changes how the brain works and even how it's structured. It involves focused attention, being mindful, or letting your thoughts flow freely. This practice activates specific brain areas linked to focus, emotional control, and self-awareness, leading to better cognitive and emotional health.

CHAPTER 2

THE CONCEPT OF PEACEFUL PRESENCE AND MEDITATION

Meditation and being in the present moment are intricately linked, as meditation often emphasises cultivating awareness of the present.

1. **Focus on Breath**

   Meditation typically involves concentrating on the breath, which helps anchor the mind to the present. By attending to the natural rhythm of inhalation and exhalation, practitioners stay grounded in the now.

2. **Mindfulness Practice**

   Meditation encourages mindfulness, which is the practice of being fully aware of the present moment. This includes observing thoughts, feelings, and sensations without judgement.

3. **Reduction of Distractions**

   Meditation reduces distractions by training the mind to return to a focal point. This enhances the ability to concentrate on the present, minimising the tendency to dwell on past regrets or future worries.

4. **Observation Without Judgement**

   Meditation teaches the skills of observing without judgement, allowing individuals to experience the present moment fully. This non-judgemental awareness aids in accepting the current reality without resistance.

5. **Enhanced Sensory Perception**

   Practising meditation can heighten sensory perception, making individuals more aware of the sounds, sights, and sensations of the present moment. This enriched sensory experience fosters a deeper connection with the now.

6. **Emotional Regulation**

   Meditation supports emotional regulation by encouraging present-moment awareness. By acknowledging and accepting emotions as they arise, individuals can respond more effectively rather than responding impulsively.

7. **Stress Reduction**

   Focusing on the present through meditation reduces stress and anxiety by shifting negative thoughts and cultivating a sense of peace and relaxation.

8. **Clarity and Insight**

   Meditation provides clarity and insight by allowing individuals to see things as they are in the present moment. This clear awareness helps in making more mindful decisions and enhances self-understanding.

9. **Detachment from Thoughts**

   Meditation promotes detachment from thoughts, seeing them as temporary phenomena rather than getting entangled in them. This practice helps individuals maintain mental balance and reduces unnecessary clutter in the mind.

By integrating these aspects into daily practice, meditation helps create a harmonious balance between mind and body, fostering a peaceful presence.

INTERNAL WISDOM - THE FOUNDATION OF MEDITATION

SELF-AWARENESS AND INTROSPECTION

Our minds are like rivers, constantly flowing with thoughts that shape our actions and behaviours. This aligns with the saying, "As we think, so we become." Just as a child learns to walk by stumbling and getting back up, or how we learn to swim by plunging into the water, sinking, and trying again, we grow through practice and persistence. This same trial-and-error approach applies to self-awareness and introspection. At first, we may feel overwhelmed by negative thoughts, but this is a natural part of the process. With consistent practice, we can train our minds to focus on the positive, breaking the cycle of negativity.

Consider the lizard, a creature that thrives even in challenging conditions. Despite its small size, it remains resilient, adapting to survive in various environments. Similarly, by nurturing positive thinking and self-awareness, we can strengthen our mental resilience, fostering a more optimistic outlook that enhances our emotional well-being.

As Ralph Waldo Emerson wisely said, "The mind, once stretched by a new idea, never returns to its original dimensions." Through introspection and self-awareness, we can expand our capacity for joy, resilience, and personal growth, just like a lizard that adapts and thrives in the face of adversity.

Introspection is a powerful tool that helps us understand our thoughts, emotions, and behaviours, which is key for personal growth and making better decisions. It allows us to manage our emotions, reduce stress, and learn from our experiences.

For example, J.K. Rowling, through self-reflection, overcame numerous rejections and hardships to create the Harry Potter series. Her journey shows how introspection can uncover strengths and guide us towards our true purpose.

Just as a lizard adapts to survive, introspection helps us adapt by uncovering underlying issues, fostering creativity, and guiding us toward personal growth. By reflecting on our values and goals, we can set meaningful objectives that align with our core principles, ultimately leading to a richer, more fulfilling life.

As a quote says, **"The more you know yourself, the more clarity there is."**

Introspection helps navigate this endless river of self-knowledge, finding peace and purpose.

Motivated by the lizard's resilience and quiet strength, I created a personal mantra: "NAVIGATING". This guiding force ignites my inner compass, empowering me to face obstacles with confidence, wisdom, and compassion. My journey has unleashed my potential, illuminating a brighter path forward.

Ready to create a foundation for self-discovery, we realised that our external world needed a refresh. We created a nurturing space with a supportive environment and gathered essential tools for our well-being.

This harmonious balance allows us to explore inner exploration and unlock our true potential.

This understanding has led me to share insights about the external and internal tools that are guiding me to navigate a peaceful presence. But before that, it's very important to know the pathway that unlocks the energy highway.

CHAPTER 3

NADIS, CHAKRAS, AND MUDRAS

(Unlocking the Energy Highway)

Imagine your body as a vibrant city, with energy flowing through its streets. In yoga, this energy is called Prana. The Nadi system is like a network of highways, distributing life force (Prana) to every corner of your being.

Nadi Highway System: Distributing Life Force

Three main highways:

1. **Sushumna Nadi: The Central Expressway**
    - Runs along the spinal cord, connecting the base (Muladhara Chakra) to the crown (Brahman Gate).
    - Balances and harmonises energy.
2. **Ida Nadi: The Cooling Highway**
    - Runs up the left side of Sushumna nadi, from Muladhara to the left nostril.
    - Associated with calmness, receptivity, and the moon's energy.

3. Pingala Nadi: The Warming Highway

- Runs up the right side of sushumna nadi, from Muladhara to the right nostril.
- Associated with activity, creativity, and the sun's energy.

Interstate Energy Exchange Hubs: Chakras

Along the Nadi highways, energy is transformed and exchanged at seven major intersections, called Chakras.

Chakras are spinning wheels of energy, transforming Prana into vital forces that nourish your body, mind, and spirit. By balancing and aligning these energy centres, you cultivate harmony and well-being.

Chakras are like the body's energetic power stations – they're in charge of your spiritual Wi-Fi! These little hubs are found in your astral body, kind of like an invisible version of you that influences everything from your creativity to your confidence, and yes, even some "superpowers".

Each chakra is connected to specific organs and systems in your physical body, including the brain, and when they're in balance, things run smoothly. Imagine them as traffic lights for your energy – when they're working, everything flows; when they're not, well, you get spiritual traffic jams!

Through meditation, you can "wake up" these chakras, helping you tune into your inner superhero, balance your energy, and unlock a sense of harmony and awareness. It's like giving your energy system a tune-up so you can cruise through life with clarity and calm!

There are seven major chakras located along the spine from the base to the crown of the head, each associated with specific colours, sounds, and emotions. They govern various aspects of our lives and have their importance. They are also connected to different endocrine glands.

1. **Root Chakra (Muladhara)**

    Placement: Base of the spine

    Importance: Grounding, stability

    Emotional Role: Safety, security, fear

    Colour: Red

    Endocrine Gland: Adrenal Glands

    Hormones: Adrenaline (stress response), Aldosterone (blood pressure)

2. **Sacral Chakra (Svadhisthana)**

    Placement: Lower abdomen

    Importance: Creativity, pleasure.

    Emotional Role: Emotions, passion, joy.

    Colour: Orange

    Hormones: Oestrogen/Testosterone (reproductive hormones)

3. **Solar Plexus Chakra (Manipura)**

    Placement: Upper abdomen

    Importance: Personal power, self-esteem

    Emotional Role: Confidence, self-worth, anger

    Colour: Yellow

    Endocrine Gland: Pancreas

    Hormones: Insulin/Glucagon (blood sugar regulation)

4. **Heart Chakra (Anahata)**

    Placement: Centre of chest

    Importance: Love, compassion.

    Emotional Role: Love, empathy, grief

Colour: Green

Endocrine Gland: Thymus

Hormones: Thymosins (immune system development)

5. **Throat Chakra (Vishuddha)**

Placement: Throat

Importance: Communication, self-expression

Emotional Role: Authenticity, truth, fear of expression

Colour: Blue

Endocrine Gland: Thyroid

Hormones: Thyroxine/Triiodothyronine (metabolism regulation)

6. **Third Eye Chakra (Ajna)**

Placement: Between eyebrows

Importance: Intuition, insight

Emotional Role: Intuition, perception, clarity.

Colour: Indigo

Endocrine Gland: Pineal Gland

Hormones: Melatonin (sleep-wake cycle regulation)

7. **Crown Chakra (Sahasrara)**

Placement: Top of head

Importance: Spiritual connection, enlightenment

Emotional Role: Spiritual awareness, connection to the universe

Colour: Violet

Endocrine Gland: Pituitary Gland

Hormones: Various (regulate other endocrine glands).

Energy Flow and Traffic Control: Mudras

Mudras are like traffic signals and signs, directing energy flow and ensuring smooth movement along the Nadi highways.

Mudras are sacred gestures that seal and direct energy within your body. They help channel Prana, quiet the mind, and connect you to your inner self.

Let us begin our body journey through Nadi highways

Brahman Gate (Crown): The ultimate destination, where Prana and Kundalini Shakti enter and exit.

Muladhara Chakra (Root): The starting point, where energy originates.

Ajna Chakra (Third Eye): A critical intersection, governing intuition and insight.

These energy highways start at the Muladhara Chakra, the foundation of your energy system. From there, they weave upwards, intersecting at strategic points influencing your physical, emotional, and mental well-being.

The Destination: Brahman Gate

The ultimate goal is to guide Kundalini Shakti, the dormant energy, upward from Muladhara to the Ajna Chakra or Brahman Gate, the crown of your energy system. This is achieved through conscious breathing, visualisation, and meditation practices.

Now, as you meditate or practice yoga, visualise these energy highways, hubs, and seals working in harmony to balance and uplift your entire being, helping in clearing energy blockages and balancing prana flow

Wake-Up Call: Start with Ajna Chakra!

Think of your chakras like a row of dominoes. To avoid a spiritual mess, tap Ajna (Third Eye) first!

Why?

1. **Detox the Basement:** Ajna purifies the lower chakras, clearing emotional junk. Imagine cleaning your closet before inviting guests over!
2. **Tame the Beast:** Awaken Ajna first, and you'll tame the karmic wild animals hiding in the lower chakras. No unexpected roar!
3. **Kundalini Kickstart:** Ajna sparks the Kundalini energy (your inner power) in the root chakra. It's like pressing the ignition button!

Start with Ajna to:

Avoid emotional turmoil

Prevent karmic chaos

Boost inner power

Don't awaken lower chakras without Ajna's guidance.

By understanding the Nadi highway system, you can optimise your energy flow, navigate life's challenges, and reach your full potential.

As we embark on this journey, let us gather the tools to illuminate our path and nurture our souls.

CHAPTER 4

EXTERNAL TOOLS: AIDS FOR ENHANCING MEDITATION

External tools are the supportive items we use to create comfort, stability, and focus during meditation. These tools help us deepen our practice and make it more enjoyable.

1. Meditation Cushion (Zafu)

A meditation cushion, or zafu, is specifically designed to provide comfort and support while sitting in meditation. Elevating the hips and allowing the knees to rest lower helps keep the spine aligned, reducing strain on the lower back and knees.

For a long time, Vikram struggled to sit comfortably on the floor for even five minutes of meditation. His posture would suffer, with his spine curving forward, and after a few minutes, he would fidget in search of comfort. This discomfort made it impossible for him to sit for longer periods. Someone recommended trying a Zafu, and it made all the difference.

Using a zafu greatly enhanced his comfort, enabling him to maintain a stable and relaxed posture for longer periods. This physical stability minimised distractions caused by discomfort, allowing for deeper mental focus.

When the spine is properly aligned, energy flows more freely through the body, nourishing every cell and organ. An open chest allows for fuller, deeper breaths, which oxygenates the body and brain, leading to increased vitality and mental clarity. Proper spinal alignment also supports the efficient functioning of internal organs, promoting healthy digestion, circulation, and overall well-being. Improved mental clarity and focus can enhance memory, mood, and intellectual function. Additionally, a well-aligned spine fosters self-esteem and confidence, providing a sense of stability and grounding. Overall, maintaining good spinal alignment is key to achieving optimal physical, mental, and emotional well-being, leading to a healthier, more vibrant life.

2. Timer or Meditation App

Meditation timers and apps can revolutionise your practice by helping you stay focused, motivated, and consistent. These tools make meditation easy and more effective, offering features that can enhance your experience:

- **Guided Meditations:** Led by experts, these provide structure and are especially helpful for beginners.
- **Customizable Timers:** Set intervals without the need to keep track of time yourself.
- **Soothing Sounds and Music:** Calm your mind and deepen your relaxation.
- **Progress Tracking and Statistics:** Monitor your growth and see how you improve over time.
- **Reminders and Notifications:** Keep your practice regular and consistent. My mobile is like a personal coach, buzzing with alarms to keep me on track as I tackle bad habits and build new, better ones. I've even got one that nudges me every 45 minutes to get up from my desk and sneak in a 2-minute power nap. It's like hitting the reset button, giving my brain a quick refresh before diving back into work with renewed energy.

Some of the top-rated meditation apps include:

- **Headspace:** Offers personalised meditation plans and progress tracking.
- **Calm:** Provides guided meditations and sleep stories to help you unwind.
- **Insight Timer:** Features timers, guided sessions, and community support.
- **Meditation Studio:** Offers a variety of meditation techniques and styles.
- **Buddhify:** Focuses on mindfulness exercises you can integrate into your daily life.

Explore these apps to find the one that best suits your meditation journey. For me, it is Insight Timer.

3. Essential Oils and Aromatherapy

Diffuse essential oils like lavender, sandalwood, or frankincense in your meditation space, or use incense sticks or cones to create a calming atmosphere as Aromatherapy enhances relaxation and focus by engaging your sense of smell. Scents like lavender promote calmness, while sandalwood offers grounding properties.

4. Meditation Journal

A meditation journal is a dedicated notebook for recording thoughts, experiences, and insights post-meditation - a powerful tool for processing your meditation practice, gaining clarity, and deepening self-understanding.

Using a meditation journal helps to:

- Track progress and note changes in mental and emotional states.
- Identify patterns and habits that may hinder growth.
- Clarify thoughts and process difficult emotions.

- Foster mindfulness and presence, enhancing focus on your journey.
- Enhance self-awareness and understanding of values and goals.

To use a meditation journal effectively:

Your meditation journal is a personal sanctuary. Be patient, kind, and compassionate with yourself as you explore your inner world. Embrace the journey and let your journal become a trusted companion on your path to greater self-awareness and inner peace.

Dedicate a few minutes post-meditation to writing. Spend a few minutes to reflect on your experiences, recording thoughts, feelings, and insights. Be honest while writing without judgement.

Explore questions for a deeper understanding and guidance. Include gratitude to cultivate a positive mindset.

5. Mindfulness Bell or Chime

A mindfulness bell or chime can be used at the beginning and end of your meditation session, or periodically during longer sessions to bring your attention back to the present moment.

Strike the bell or chime gently to produce a clear, resonant sound. Focus on the sound as it fades, allowing it to centre your mind.

The sound of the bell or chime acts as an auditory anchor, helping you to return to your focus if your mind starts to wander. It also marks the transition into and out of meditation, creating a ritualistic aspect that enhances mindfulness.

6. WATER AND FOOD

"Water and food are essential for our physical well-being; they can also be considered external tools that lay the groundwork for a successful meditation practice."

A nourishing diet and proper hydration help calm the mind, reduce physical discomfort, and increase focus, making it easier to settle into a meditative state. Although eating and drinking are not meditation practices themselves, they serve as preparatory steps that enable us to engage in meditation with greater clarity and comfort.

Water

Water possesses life-giving properties and can profoundly enhance our well-being. Given that our bodies are composed of approximately 70% water.

Connecting Solar Plexus Meditation with Water

The solar plexus, or Manipura chakra, is like the command centre of your body, located just below your ribcage. Imagine it as the powerhouse that keeps everything running smoothly—whether it's managing digestion, distributing energy, handling stress, or regulating emotions and hormones. This vital energy centre is like your body's multitasking superhero, ensuring everything stays in balance and harmony.

Now, imagine your solar plexus as a peaceful lake. When life gets stressful, that calm lake can turn into a chaotic whirlpool, leaving you feeling all sorts of frazzled. But don't worry! With a bit of meditation, you can soothe those choppy waters, turning that wild whirlpool back into a serene, glassy surface that reflects clarity and calmness.

So, when the world feels like it's spinning out of control, just remember to tap into your inner superhero (solar plexus), give it some tender loving care with meditation, nurture it with mindfulness and relaxation, and watch those waters settle back into peaceful tranquillity.

The combination of Solar Plexus meditation or Manipura - a third chakra and water can create a powerful practice that enhances the benefits of both elements. Water, symbolising purification and emotional balance, can amplify the energy of the Solar Plexus Chakra, boosting self-esteem, self-control, and overall energy levels.

Steps to Integrate Solar Plexus Meditation with Water

1. **Preparation:**
   - Find a quiet and comfortable place a bowl of water in front of you during your meditation.
2. **Set an Intention:**
   - Begin with a clear intention such as, "I intend to empower and cleanse my Solar Plexus Chakra with the energy of water."
3. **Begin with Deep Breathing:**
   - Sit comfortably with your spine straight. Close your eyes and take several deep breaths. Inhale deeply through your nose, allowing your abdomen to expand, and exhale slowly through your mouth.
4. **Focus on the Solar Plexus Chakra:**
   - Direct your attention to the area just above your navel. Visualise a bright, golden-yellow light glowing and becoming brighter and more vibrant with each breath.
5. **Visualization with Water: Place your hands around the bowl (without touching the bowl) and visualize the golden light flowing into the water, charging it with energy and positivity.**
6. **Affirmations: Repeat affirmations such as**
   - "I am confident and strong."
   - "I radiate positive energy."
   - "I am in control of my life."

   You can have your affirmations.

7. Drinking Energised Water

After meditation, drink the energised water slowly, imagining the positive energy spreading throughout your body.

8. Express Gratitude

Conclude with gratitude for the energy and water, such as, "Thank you for the empowerment and clarity this practice has brought me."

Benefits of Combining Solar Plexus Meditation with Water

1. Enhanced Energy Flow:

- Water amplifies the energy generated from the Solar Plexus Chakra, making meditation more potent

2. Improved Emotional Stability:

- The calming properties of water can help balance emotions, making it easier to focus on personal empowerment and confidence.

3. Increased Clarity and Purification:

- Water's cleansing properties can help remove blockages from the Solar Plexus Chakra, allowing for clearer and more powerful energy flow and restoring the balance to the energy centres (chakras).

4. Boosted Physical Well-being:

- Drinking energised water can enhance your overall physical health by promoting better hydration and aiding in the body's natural healing processes. It boosts energy levels and vitality.

5. Deepened Spiritual Connection:

- Integrating water into your meditation practice can deepen your connection to the natural elements and enhance your overall spiritual well-being.

Meditating on the solar plexus with the transparent glass of water became a powerful tool for Vikram during his tough times. His mind found strength and clarity. This practice allowed him to manage pain with calmness, building resilience and an unwavering hope for survival. Each morning, the first thing we did was fill a transparent glass with water and follow the solar plexus meditation process, using affirmations and mantras to start the day with positive energy. We began to truly live in the moment, cherishing our time together and feeling deeply blessed that I could be there for him when he needed me most.

Over time, I transformed from a constantly anxious person into a strong woman who learned to accept situations as they are and trust the universe. Months of dedicated practice helped me embrace my fate and believe that God has a plan for the best. This newfound belief brought me immense strength and peace, allowing me to face each day calmly and focus on the present rather than worrying about the future.

By combining the Solar Plexus meditation with the natural properties of water, you can create a powerful practice that boosts personal empowerment.

FOOD

In traditional Indian dietary classifications, foods are categorised into three types: Sattvic, Rajasic, and Tamasic, each influencing the body and mind differently.

Sattvic Food: Sattvic food, meaning purity and harmony in Sanskrit, includes fresh, organic, and natural foods such as fruits, vegetables, whole grains, nuts, seeds, and dairy products like milk and ghee. This diet is known to enhance mental clarity, emotional stability, and physical health, making it ideal for meditation. Sattvic foods are light and nourishing, promoting a calm and serene mind essential for deep meditative states. They ensure energy is efficiently used, reducing stress and anxiety, and aligning the body and mind for a more effective meditation practice.

Rajasic Food: Rajasic foods are stimulating and increase activity and restlessness. This category includes spicy foods like chillies and pepper, caffeinated beverages like coffee and tea, salty snacks such as chips and pretzels, and oily, fried foods including fast food. While these foods can energise, they also lead to overstimulation, increasing stress and anxiety levels.

Tamasic Food: Tamasic foods are considered dulling or lethargy-inducing. They include processed foods like packaged snacks, stale or leftover foods, heavy meats such as red meat and pork, and alcohol. These foods can reduce vitality and induce lethargy, making them less suitable for maintaining a balanced and alert state of mind.

Sattvic Food and Meditation: Combining a sattvic diet with meditation creates a conducive environment for achieving deep meditative states. Sattvic foods nourish without causing heaviness, keeping the mind alert and focused. They promote a balanced digestive system, ensuring energy isn't diverted to digestion. This diet helps reduce stress and anxiety, fostering inner peace and tranquillity, which are crucial for meditation. The purity of sattvic foods aligns with the meditative goal of attaining pure consciousness and spiritual enlightenment, leading to a balanced, peaceful, enlightened life.

The food we consume fuels our physical well-being and catalyses our mental and emotional harmony. A diet rich in vibrant, rainbow-coloured, and sattvic ingredients awakens inner vitality, clarifies the mind, and uplifts the spirit, fostering a holistic approach to well-being.

Acharya Mahapragyaji believed that a person who controls their diet will stay healthy, young, and active. He knew that if he wanted to study deep spiritual texts and meditate intensely, he needed to follow a simple, balanced diet. This way, his body wouldn't waste energy on digestion. His thoughts on food were very clear. He understood that food nourishes the body, so he chose to eat only what would benefit both his mind and heart, rather than foods that would strain his liver and intestines.

In one of his satsangs, Acharya Mahapragyaji said that the best food is the kind that boosts your energy, repairs damaged tissues, helps remove toxins, and makes you feel lighter and happier.

Meditation for Mindful Eating:

1. **Set an Intention**: Before you begin eating, take a moment to set a mindful intention. This can help you focus on the present moment and appreciate the nourishment you are about to receive.
2. **Create a Calm Environment**: Eat in a quiet, distraction-free space to fully engage with your meal.
3. **Take Deep Breaths**: Start your meal by taking a few deep breaths. This helps to calm your mind and body, preparing you for a mindful eating experience.
4. **Engage Your Senses**: Notice the colours, textures, and aromas of food. Engaging all your senses can enhance the eating experience and promote gratitude for the food.
5. **Be Present with Each Bite**: Focus on eating. Chew each bite slowly and thoroughly. Pay attention to how the food feels in your mouth, the taste, and how your body responds to it.
6. **Listen to Your Body:** Tune into your hunger and fullness signals. Aim to eat until you feel satisfied, not overly full, and stop when you feel comfortably satiated.
7. **Reflect on Your Eating Experience:** After eating, take a moment to notice any physical or emotional responses to your meal. Reflect on how the food made you feel and your mindful eating practice.

8. **Express Gratitude:** Show gratitude for your food by acknowledging the journey it took to reach your plate and the nourishment it provides. Thank everyone involved in bringing the food to you.
9. **Practice Regularly:** Make mindful eating a regular part of your routine. Consistent practice can enhance your relationship with food, improve digestion, and promote overall well-being.

By integrating these techniques into your eating habits, you can create a more mindful and enjoyable eating experience that benefits both your body and mind.

The external path has prepared us for the inner journey.

Now, let us venture forth into the depths of our hearts and minds.

CHAPTER 5

INTERNAL TOOLS NAVIGATING PEACEFUL PRESENCE

"Like a desert reptile basking in the sun's warm light,
We too can find our inner peace and let our spirits take flight.
With scales of protection and eyes that see beyond,
We navigate life's challenges and find our inner bond.

In the stillness of the desert, we find our quiet core,
A place of refuge, where love and calm await in store.
Like the lizard's gentle gaze, we focus on our way,
And trust the universe to guide us, come what may.

With each breath, we shed our fears, like a reptile sheds its skin,
And emerge anew, reborn, with a heart that's light within.
May we embrace our inner strength and find our peaceful nest,
Like the desert lizard, who knows its true self, and finds its rest."

Healthy habits and internal tools can help us navigate life's challenges with greater ease and confidence. Just as a lizard navigates through the desert with its keen senses and adaptability, we too can develop our inner guidance system. By utilising techniques like visualisation, breathwork, and affirmations, we can stay focused and calm, even in turbulent times.

These internal tools serve as beacons, shining brightly like a lighthouse in the darkness, guiding us toward tranquillity and clarity. As we practice and incorporate them into our daily lives, we become more resilient, like a lizard's scales protecting it from the harsh desert environment.

By trusting our heart's way and embracing our inner strength, we can adapt and thrive in life's shifting sands. Just as a lizard finds its peaceful nest, we too can discover our serene presence, where love and calm await. May we embody the lizard's gentle gaze and focused intent, trusting the universe to guide us as we navigate life's journey.

Simply knowing words isn't enough to achieve self-discovery. You must first admit what you don't know and then use the right techniques to gain a deeper understanding of yourself.

Imagine trying to navigate a new city without a map or GPS. You might know the names of some streets and landmarks, but you won't truly understand the layout until you acknowledge your confusion and use a reliable guide to find your way. Similarly, self-discovery requires more than just familiarising yourself with spiritual concepts – it demands humility, recognition of your limitations, and a willingness to explore your inner world using effective methods.

Embark on life's journey using the acronym NAVIGATING to guide you. Nurture your mind, anchor in the present, visualise peace, Introspect regularly, ground yourself, affirm positively, trust the process, integrate daily, navigate challenges, and guide your way to tranquillity and clarity.

N - NOW

A - AWARENESS

V - VISUALIZATION

I - INTUITION

G - GRATITUDE

A - AFFIRMATION

T - TRANSFORMATION

I - INTEGRITY

N - NOURISHMENT

G - GROUNDING

N - NOW

Embracing the present moment is transformative, much like how a lizard instinctively adapts to its surroundings. When we focus on the *now*, we unlock our potential, enhancing mindfulness and deepening our meditation practice. The lizard's ability to stay attuned to its environment reminds us of the importance of being fully present.

When the primary earner of a family falls ill, their concern naturally shifts from their own health to the well-being of their family, which can lead to overwhelming anxiety and a loss of focus on the present. Vikram found himself caught in this cycle of fear and stress, which only compounded his health issues.

However, an unlikely teacher—a simple lizard—offered him a new perspective. Observing the lizard's calm, present-focused existence inspired Vikram to change his approach. Rather than fretting about the future, he began to adopt the lizard's way of responding to its environment - calmly, without fear of what might happen next.

This newfound insight motivated Vikram to seek techniques for staying grounded in the present, such as breath control and mindfulness through Preksha Dhyan guided meditation. These practices became key to helping him manage his situation with clarity and inner peace.

We both embraced these techniques, integrating them with the wisdom I had gained from Jain monks and nuns, to deepen our practice of being fully present. Over time, these practices, which I will explain in the following chapters, became our tools for navigating life's challenges with serenity and clarity. Instead of being weighed down by fear and anxiety, we learned to approach each situation with a calm, composed mind, empowering us to face difficulties with resilience and grace.

By connecting with the present through mindful breathing, we anchor ourselves in reality, dissolving distractions and fostering clarity. This state of awareness is not just the essence of meditation but also a path to inner peace and personal growth. As Eckhart Tolle wisely notes, "Realise deeply that the present moment is all you ever have."

When we fully engage our senses, we escape the chaos of overthinking, similar to how a lizard finds calm amidst its surroundings. This mindful presence allows us to experience life more vividly, making even the simplest tasks more enjoyable and less overwhelming.

The present moment is the gateway to freedom. Emotions emerge where the mind and body intersect. A thought of being threatened triggers a bodily response, such as contraction, recognised as fear. If you struggle to feel your emotions, direct your attention to your body's inner energy field—sense your body from within. The most effective way to achieve this connection is through mindful breathing, enhancing awareness of both your body and emotions, leading to a deeper sense of inner calm and liberation.

When overwhelmed with problems, there's no space for new ideas or solutions. It's crucial to create room to discover the essence of your life beneath current situations. Engage your senses fully. Be present without overthinking. Simply observe – notice the light, shapes, colours, and textures around you. Acknowledge the silent presence of everything. Pay attention to the space that allows all things to exist. Listen to sounds without judgement, noticing the silence underneath. Touch objects and recognise their existence. Observe the rhythm of your breath, feeling the air move in and out, sensing the life energy within your body. Embrace everything as it is, both inside and outside of you, immersing yourself deeply in the present moment.

By doing this, you leave behind the dull world of mental abstractions and time, escaping the mind's chaos, which drains your energy and harms your well-being. You awaken from the dream of time into the vividness of the present.

Consider whether there's joy, ease, and lightness in your actions. If not, it means time is obscuring the present moment, making life seem like a burden. For example, if you're working on a project and feel stressed, it's a sign you're not fully present. Take a moment to breathe deeply, feel your surroundings, and reconnect with the present. This shift can make tasks more enjoyable and less overwhelming.

By practising mindful breathing and being present, you cultivate awareness that enriches your meditation and daily life, guiding you towards a path of serenity and self-discovery.

A - AWARENESS

Awareness Towards the Body in Meditation and Mindfulness plays a fundamental role in achieving a balanced mental and physical state. By focusing on the body, we foster a deep connection between the mind and physical sensations, promoting greater relaxation, presence, and emotional regulation. Here's how different techniques can guide us in this practice:

1. **Somatic Awareness:**

   Becoming consciously aware of your bodily sensations, movements, and posture bridges the gap between the mind and body. This awareness helps you notice how physical sensations influence your emotions and thoughts. For instance, tension in your shoulders might indicate stress. By acknowledging these sensations without judgement, you can release physical discomfort and foster mental clarity.

2. **Body Scan Technique:**

   This involves mentally scanning different parts of your body from head to toe, bringing attention to each one. By doing so, you promote relaxation and reduce tension. It allows you to systematically become aware of any tightness or discomfort, releasing it with each breath.

3. **Embodiment:**

   Emotions often manifest physically before we're even consciously aware of them. Recognising how your body reacts to feelings like stress or joy can help manage those emotions effectively. By practising embodiment, you can learn to regulate your emotional state, reducing the tendency to react impulsively.

4. **Mindful Movement:**

   Practices like yoga or deep breathing exercises integrate body awareness with gentle movements. These techniques bring mindfulness into your daily life, enhancing your connection to the present moment and reducing distractions.

Preksha Meditation and Body Awareness:

Acharya Mahapragya, a respected Jain monk, emphasised the use of body scanning in his teachings on Preksha Meditation. This method teaches us to observe bodily sensations with neutrality, cultivating a deeper understanding of the body-mind connection.

- **Focusing on Body Parts:** In Preksha Meditation, attention is systematically directed to different areas of the body. This fosters relaxation and mindfulness, easing physical and mental tension.

When we progressively move our awareness through different parts of the body, it does more than just induce physical relaxation. It acts like a mental “clean-up,” clearing the nerve pathways connected to both physical actions and sensory input, essentially rebooting the system. By paying attention to each area, we also stimulate the brain, almost like running a mental scan from the inside out.

For instance, imagine you’re doing a **body scan meditation**. You start at your toes, consciously relaxing them, and slowly move upwards to your legs and head. Not only does this help release tension, but it also activates neural pathways, improving both physical control and mental clarity. As you become more attuned to your body, you’re effectively sending signals to your brain that you’re in a relaxed, focused state, which in turn enhances your overall mindfulness.

This focused awareness helps reduce stress and anxiety, leaving you both physically relaxed and mentally clear, much like a computer reset, allowing both the mind and body to function in harmony.

- **Observing Sensations:** Observing without attachment helps practitioners understand how emotions manifest physically, promoting emotional stability and self-awareness.
- **Breath Awareness:** By connecting breath with bodily awareness, the mind becomes anchored in the present moment, heightening meditation's impact.

Connecting to the Present Moment:

1. Buddha: "The secret of health for both mind and body is not to mourn for the past, worry about the future, or anticipate troubles, but to live in the present moment wisely and earnestly."
2. Zen Proverb: "You should meditate for twenty minutes every day—unless you're too busy. Then you should sit for an hour."

By becoming mindful of your body, you strengthen the link between your physical sensations and emotional well-being, enriching your meditation practice. Through the wisdom of techniques like body scanning and mindful movement, you can unlock deeper relaxation, enhance focus, and live with greater presence and balance.

V - FOR VISUALISATION

A POWERFUL TOOL FOR SHAPING REALITY

Visualisation is the powerful practice of creating vivid mental images to shape reality, cultivate positivity, and manifest desires. **Buddha quotes "The mind is everything. What you think, you become."**

Visualisation isn't just about seeing an image or having a thought – it's the emotion behind it that creates true attraction. If you constantly project your feelings into the future, they will stay there. Instead, connect those feelings with the present moment. When you truly feel as if your desired outcome is happening now, it becomes an open doorway for the universe to start bringing it into your reality.

This way, the power of the universe begins to align with your intention, allowing your visualised goals to manifest in the present, rather than staying in the distant future.

Effective visualisation involves:

- **Clarity:** Vividly imagining specific details and outcomes.
- **Emotional connection**: Infusing mental images with positive emotions
- **Consistency**: Regularly practising visualisation to reinforce mental patterns
- **Belief**: Trusting in the power of visualisation to shape reality.

When you visualise, focus on a clear image of your desired outcome and keep that picture steady in your mind. Trust in the power of your imagination, knowing that the universe will align its forces to help you achieve your goal.

For example, imagine you're aiming for a promotion at work. Picture yourself confidently sitting in your new office, tackling projects with ease, and celebrating your success. As you hold onto that vision with faith, your actions and decisions begin aligning with that goal. Slowly but surely, opportunities arise – whether it's impressing your boss with an idea or networking with the right people. The universe responds to your clarity and belief, guiding you towards that result.

Olympic athlete Jim Thorpe, a world-class runner and expert visualiser, used visualization to overcome challenges with his javelin throws before the 1912 Stockholm Olympics. By vividly imagining himself throwing the javelin with perfect technique and infusing the mental image with confidence, Thorpe was able to break his record and set a new world record the next day. This example demonstrates how visualization can reprogram the mind and body for elite performance.

Some techniques of visualisation:

1. **Mind's Eye Visualization**: Close your eyes and imagine yourself in a specific scenario, using all your senses to create a vivid mental picture. Visualise yourself achieving your goals, overcoming challenges, or experiencing a desired outcome.
2. **Creative Visualization:** Picture your ideal life, career, relationships, and surroundings. This technique helps to manifest your desires by tapping into your creative potential.
3. **Guided Visualization:** Use a guided audio recording to lead you through a visualization process. This technique helps you relax, focus, and access your subconscious mind, making it easier to visualise and manifest your goals.
4. **Visualisation with Emotion:** This technique involves connecting with your emotions while visualising. When combined with strong, positive emotions like excitement, joy, or confidence, this technique significantly impacts the subconscious. By emotionally engaging with your visualizations, you:

- Amplify the impact on your subconscious mind.
- Boost motivation and commitment to your goals.
- Increase the likelihood of manifesting your desires

Emotions serve as the driving force behind visualization, turning abstract images into a potent reality-shaping tool. To maximise the effectiveness of visualisation with emotion, use pre-use present-tense affirmations such as "I am" instead of "I will be."

Imagine yourself standing on a beach at sunset, feeling the warm sand beneath your feet and the gentle ocean breeze on your skin. Visualise the vibrant colours of the sky, the soothing sound of the waves, and the salty aroma of the sea.

We all have more power and potential than we often realise, and visualisation is one of the strongest abilities we possess. Everyone visualises, whether they are aware of it or not, and this is one of the key secrets to success. The only thing that can stop your vision from becoming reality is the very power that created it in the first place – you.

As you immerse yourself in this emotional visualization, your subconscious mind starts to believe that this feeling of success is real. It begins to rewire your thoughts, behaviours, and actions to align with the desired outcome, unlock creativity, tap into innovative ideas, build resilience, and cultivate a growth mindset by embracing the challenges and growing from them. The emotional connection amplifies the visualization, making it more potent and effective in manifesting your goals.

Individuals can achieve a wide range of benefits by harnessing the mind's incredible ability to create mental scenarios.

I - INTUITION

Intuition is an innate ability to understand or know something without conscious reasoning. Often described as a "gut feeling" or inner voice, intuition guides decisions and actions, drawing on past experiences, emotions, and subconscious knowledge. For instance, you might instinctively sense danger or feel a connection with someone without clear evidence. This immediate, holistic insight plays a crucial role in creativity, problem-solving, and relationships, helping you navigate life's complexities with greater ease and confidence.

Trusting your intuition is a powerful way to make decisions aligned with your true self. When decisions and actions resonate with our true selves, they feel right at a fundamental level. This resonance means that our choices are in tune with our authentic identity, not influenced by external pressures or expectations. It's about being genuine, making decisions that feel true to who we are rather than conforming to what others might expect of us. There's no internal conflict or doubt, just a calm certainty that we are on the right path. This harmony is essential for overall well-being, as it fosters contentment and reduces the inner turmoil that often comes with decision-making.

Steve Jobs' journey as the co-founder of Apple Inc. was deeply influenced by his reliance on intuition. He made the bold decision to drop out of college and study calligraphy, driven by a gut feeling rather than logical reasoning. This unconventional decision, guided purely by intuition, eventually influenced the elegant typography and design principles that became hallmarks of Apple's products. Jobs' willingness to follow his inner guidance not only shaped the aesthetic of the Macintosh computer but also set a new standard in product design, demonstrating how intuition can lead to profound and unexpected innovation.

Another example is Malala Yousafzai, the Pakistani activist for female education and the youngest Nobel Prize laureate.

Despite the immense danger and opposition she faced, Malala trusted her inner voice, which told her that advocating for girls' education was the right thing to do. Her unwavering belief in her cause, guided by her intuition, not only survived a life-threatening attack but also became a global symbol of courage and justice. Malala's story illustrates how intuition can guide individuals to act with integrity and impact the world positively.

Intuition also plays a crucial role in everyday decision-making. For instance, someone might feel an inexplicable urge to take a different route to work one day, only to discover later that they avoided a major traffic accident. This kind of intuitive guidance helps individuals avoid potential harm and make choices that enhance their well-being.

Moreover, intuition can help in personal relationships. By trusting your inner voice, you can better understand and navigate complex emotional landscapes. For example, you might sense that a friend needs support before they even express it. Acting on this intuition can strengthen your bond and provide timely assistance, fostering deeper connections and mutual understanding.

Trusting intuition requires mindfulness - being fully aware and present in the moment. When we are mindful, we can better hear and trust our inner voice. This presence allows us to tap into our intuition more clearly, without the noise of distractions or overthinking. It's about slowing down, listening to our instincts, and allowing our inner wisdom to guide us.

In essence, intuition acts as a compass. Just as a compass provides direction, intuition guides us towards decisions and actions that align with our true selves. It's an internal sense of direction that helps us navigate life's complexities without needing explicit evidence or logical reasoning. This compass, however, isn't just about pointing us in the right direction—it's about ensuring that the direction we take is in harmony with who we truly are, our core values, and our deepest desires.

G - GRATITUDE

THE GATEWAY TO FORGIVENESS

Gratitude is the golden thread that weaves together the tapestry of our lives, showing us the beauty around us. BK Shibani says, "Gratitude is the sweetest fragrance that emanates from the flowers of appreciation, filling our hearts with joy, humility, and happiness."

Forgiveness: The Liberation of the Soul

Forgiveness is like a refreshing rain that soothes our souls, bringing us peace and freedom. It's the brave act of letting go of anger, hurt, and resentment and choosing to understand and care for others instead.

Eckhart Tolle, in *The Power of Now*, underscores the deep link between forgiveness and gratitude, revealing how these two concepts work together to create inner peace. He suggests that forgiveness is not merely about releasing someone else from blame but about freeing ourselves from the burden of past grievances. By letting go of anger and resentment, we stop living in the shadow of past hurts, which opens up the possibility of truly experiencing the present moment.

Forgiveness is like opening a door that has long been shut, allowing the fresh air of gratitude to enter our lives. When we forgive, we make space within ourselves to appreciate the present, acknowledging the good that exists around us. Tolle points out that this act of forgiveness doesn't just benefit those we forgive—it's primarily for our liberation. It helps us to stop dwelling on what was and start embracing what is, which naturally leads to feelings of gratitude.

In simple terms, Tolle's message is about shifting our focus from the pain of the past to the richness of the present. When we forgive, we aren't just letting go of the past; we are actively choosing to live more fully in the present. This choice to live in the now is where gratitude blossoms, turning our attention to the beauty and blessings that are already part of our lives. By doing this, we transform our perspective, allowing gratitude to fill the spaces once occupied by negativity, thereby enriching our lives with positivity and peace.

Louise Hay, an influential author and speaker, offers profound perspectives on gratitude and forgiveness:

- "Gratitude is a transformative practice that can shift your mindset and invite more positivity into your life."
- "By concentrating on the blessings you have rather than what you lack, you open the door to greater abundance."
- "Forgiveness is a liberating gift you give yourself, allowing you to release the emotional burdens that hinder your growth."
- "There is a deep connection between gratitude and forgiveness. When you embrace gratitude, it becomes easier to forgive, and in forgiving, you naturally find more to be grateful for."

Hay emphasises that the foundation of true gratitude and forgiveness lies in the love and acceptance of oneself.

Rhonda Byrne, the author of *The Secret,* emphasises the significance of gratitude and forgiveness in enhancing visualisation techniques. She explains that cultivating gratitude aligns our energy with positivity, allowing us to focus on what we want to create in our lives. By practising gratitude, we raise our vibrational frequency, making it easier to visualise and attract our desires. Forgiveness, on the other hand, releases negative energy and emotions, clearing the mind and heart for a clearer visualisation practice. When we forgive, we let go of resistance and open ourselves to receiving our desires. Byrne suggests that by combining gratitude and forgiveness with visualisation, we can manifest our dreams more effectively. She recommends starting each day with gratitude and forgiveness, followed by focused visualisation, to harness the power of the Law of Attraction. By doing so, we can tap into the universe's abundance and bring our desires into reality.

Here are some techniques to cultivate gratitude habits.

1. Gratitude Journal: Write down three things you're thankful for each day before bed.
2. Morning Gratitude: Start your day by sharing three things you're grateful for with a friend or family member.
3. Gratitude Jar: Write down things you're thankful for on slips of paper and put them in a jar. Read them when you need a boost.
4. Share Your Gratitude: Express thanks to someone you appreciate, whether in person, via text, or email.
5. Mindful Moments: Take a few minutes each day to focus on your breath and reflect on the good things in your life.
6. Gratitude Letter: Write a heartfelt letter to someone who has made a positive impact in your life (even if you don't intend to send it).
7. Daily Reflection: Take a minute...

A gratitude journal is a transformative tool that cultivates a profound sense of appreciation and positivity in our lives. By dedicating a few minutes each day to writing down three to five things we are thankful for, we begin to shift our focus from what's lacking to what we already have. This simple yet powerful practice rewires our brains to recognise the abundance of blessings in our lives, no matter how small they may seem. As we reflect on the good things, we start to notice a profound impact on our well-being, relationships, and outlook. Gratitude journals have been shown to increase happiness, reduce stress and anxiety, and foster deeper connections with others.

A - AFFIRMATION AND MANTRAS

Affirmations and mantras are powerful tools used to focus the mind, promote positive thinking, and foster inner peace. While they share similarities, such as being repeated phrases or statements, they serve different purposes and originate from different cultural and spiritual traditions.

Affirmations are positive statements that are consciously crafted to challenge and overcome self-sabotaging and negative thoughts. They are used in various aspects of self-improvement, personal growth, and mental health. The idea behind affirmations is rooted in the belief that positive thinking can manifest positive results in one's life. For example, repeating statements like "I am confident and capable" or "I attract success and abundance" can help individuals build self-esteem, reduce stress, and create a positive mindset. Louise Hay, a renowned author and motivational speaker, popularised affirmations in her works, encouraging people to use them to improve their lives and well-being.

Mantras, on the other hand, have deep spiritual and historical significance, particularly in Eastern traditions such as Hinduism, Jainism, and Buddhism.

A mantra is a word or symbol that embodies a particular view of the divine and the universe. Mantras hold immense power and are often bestowed upon disciples by enlightened teachers who understand the profound significance of the syllables. When a mantra is given to a disciple by an illumined teacher, it transforms into a living seed. The teacher, through their spiritual power, infuses life into the mantra and simultaneously awakens the dormant spiritual energies within the disciple. This process is the essence of the teacher's initiation.

The belief is that while chanting a mantra, one should visualise the deity associated with that mantra. It is also said that the beneficial effects of japa (mantra chanting) are realised only after chanting the mantra a hundred thousand times. This practice requires devotion, consistency, and patience, as the repetitive chanting helps to deepen the disciple's spiritual connection and brings about transformative changes.

For instance, in Hinduism, the mantra "Om Namah Shivaya" is often chanted with the visualization of Lord Shiva. The disciple is encouraged to focus on Shiva's form, attributes, and energy. Over time, this practice can lead to a deeper spiritual awakening and a sense of unity with the divine.

Some of the powerful mantras:

Om Mantra

The Om Mantra, also known as the Pranava Mantra, is considered the primordial sound and the most sacred syllable in Hinduism, Buddhism, and Jainism. It represents the ultimate reality, the universe, and the divine. The sound "Om" comprises three phonetic components: "A", "U", and "M", symbolising the creation, preservation, and dissolution of the universe. Chanting Om helps in calming the mind, reducing stress, and fostering a deep sense of connection with the universe. It is believed to resonate within the body, promoting physical and mental healing, and enhancing spiritual growth.

Sadguru's Teaching on the AUM Mantra and Its Connection to Chakras and Body Parts

Sadhguru, a renowned spiritual teacher, emphasises the profound impact of chanting the AUM mantra on an individual's physical, mental, and spiritual well-being. The mantra AUM is not just a sound but a representation of the entire universe and the consciousness that underlies it. Each component of AUM (A, U, M) corresponds to different aspects of the body and the energy system, particularly the chakras.

Breakdown of AUM:

1. "A" Sound:
   - Chakra: Corresponds to the Manipura (Solar Plexus) Chakra.
   - Body Part: Resonates with the lower abdomen.
   - Function: The "A" sound is guttural, originating from the base of the throat. It represents the creation aspect of the universe and stimulates the Manipura chakra, which governs willpower and energy distribution in the body. Chanting "A" energises and activates the lower abdomen, enhancing digestion and vitality.
2. "U" Sound:
   - Chakra: Corresponds to the Anahata (Heart) Chakra.
   - Body Part: Resonates through the chest.
   - Function: The "U" sound is pronounced from the middle of the vocal tract, transitioning from the back of the mouth. It symbolises the preservation aspect of the universe and connects deeply with the heart chakra, which is the centre of love and compassion. Chanting "U" expands the chest and heart area, promoting emotional balance and well-being.
3. "M" Sound:
   - Chakra: Corresponds to the Ajna (Third Eye) Chakra.
   - Body Part: Resonates in the head.
   - Function: The "M" sound is created by closing the lips, resulting in a humming vibration that resonates in the head. It represents the dissolution aspect of the universe and stimulates the ajna chakra, the seat of intuition and wisdom. Chanting "M" calms the mind and enhances mental clarity and focus.

Integration of AUM with the Entire Chakra System:

- The act of chanting AUM is holistic, as it traverses through different chakras and body parts, creating a balance of energies within the system.
- Chanting Sequence: Starting from the lower abdomen (A), moving up through the chest (U), and finally resonating in the head (M), the mantra travels through the main energy centres, harmonising and aligning them.
- Energetic Flow: This sequence not only activates specific chakras but also ensures a smooth flow of prana (life energy) throughout the body, connecting the physical, emotional, and spiritual aspects of a person.

Benefits of AUM Chanting:

1. Physical Health:
    - Enhances respiratory function through controlled breathing.
    - Stimulates and balances the endocrine system via chakra activation.
    - Promotes better digestion and energy distribution in the body.
2. Emotional Balance:
    - Releases pent-up emotions and stress through heart chakra activation.
    - Cultivates a sense of inner peace and emotional stability.
3. Mental Clarity:
    - Calms the mind and reduces mental clutter.
    - Enhances focus, concentration, and intuitive abilities.
4. Spiritual Growth:
    - Facilitates a deeper connection with the universal consciousness.

- Awakens and strengthens latent spiritual potential.

Practical Application:

- Daily Practice: Incorporating AUM chanting into daily meditation can significantly enhance overall well-being.
- Focused Sessions: During meditation, focus on each component of AUM, visualising the corresponding chakra and body part, feeling the vibrations and their effects.

The transformative power of the ancient mantra 'Aum' taught by Sadguru had a profound impact on Vikram's well-being. As he embraced its soothing vibrations, his mind quieted, and his body responded with remarkable resilience. The infection that had taken hold of his lungs began to dissipate, making way for enhanced respiratory function and a symphony of hormonal balance. This transformative experience not only healed his physical body but also nourished his spirit.

Gayatri Mantra:

ॐ भूर्भुवः स्वः

तत्सवितुर्वरेण्यं

भर्गो देवस्य धीमहि

धियो यो नः प्रचोदयात्

English Transliteration:

Om Bhur Bhuvah Svah

Tat Savitur Varenyam

Bhargo Devasya Dhimahi.

Dhiyo Yo Nah Prachodayat

Meaning:

- Om: The primordial sound and symbol of the universal consciousness.
- Bhur: The physical realm.

- Bhuvah: The mental realm.
- Svah: The spiritual realm.
- Tat: That (referring to God or the ultimate reality).
- Savitur: The Sun or the divine light.
- Varenyam: Adorable, worthy of worship.
- Bhargo: Divine radiance.
- Devasya: Of the divine.
- Dhimahi: We meditate upon.
- Dhiyo: Intellects.
- Yo: Who.
- Nah: Our.
- Prachodayat: Enlighten, inspire.

Full Translation:

"We meditate on the divine light of the adorable sun of spiritual consciousness. May it illuminate our minds and inspire our intellects."

The Gayatri Mantra is one of the most revered and powerful mantras in Hinduism. It is a Vedic mantra dedicated to Savitar, the sun deity, and it seeks to inspire wisdom and enlightenment. The mantra is composed of twenty-four syllables and is found in the Rigveda. The Gayatri Mantra is recited to invoke the divine light and to foster a higher state of consciousness. Regular chanting of the Gayatri Mantra is believed to bring spiritual and material benefits, promoting clarity of thought, inner peace, and overall well-being. It serves as a guide to right living and a tool for personal transformation.

After waking up, after answering the calls of nature and cleansing your body, ensure that your mind remains focused and does not wander. Devote your time to performing the morning japa, which is the GAYATRI mantra, with utmost sincerity. Stand on your feet and recite the mantra very slowly and deliberately.

According to the Vedas, it is recommended to chant the Gayatri Mantra at both dawn and dusk, standing in water, and if there is no water, then taking water in your palm while facing the Sun. In the morning, face eastward, and in the evening, turn westward. **This sacred mantra should never be recited after sunset.**

NAMASKAR MANTRA:

In Jainism, the Namaskar Mantra is a revered prayer that honours enlightened beings and seeks their guidance. It is also known as the Navkar Mantra or Namokar Mantra.

णमो अरिहंताणं

णमो सिद्धाणं

णमो आयरियाणं

णमो उवज्झायाणं

णमो लोए सव्व साहुणं

English Translation:

I bow to the enlightened beings (Arihants).

I bow to the liberated souls (Siddhas).

I bow to the spiritual leaders (Acharyas).

I bow to the spiritual teachers (Upadhyayas).

I bow to all the monks and nuns (Sadhus and Sadhvis).

The Namaskar Mantra honours the qualities of:

- Arihants (Conquerors): Embodiment of self-control, wisdom, and liberation
- Siddhas (Liberated Souls): Represent perfect detachment, bliss, and ultimate freedom.
- Acharyas (Spiritual Leaders): Exemplify guidance, wisdom, and spiritual growth.

- Upadhyayas (Spiritual Teachers): Embody knowledge, compassion, and selflessness.
- Sadhus and Sadhvis (Monks and Nuns): Represent renunciation, austerity, and spiritual discipline.

By worshipping these qualities, Jains aspire to cultivate them within themselves, striving for spiritual growth, self-realisation, and ultimate liberation. This approach focuses on emulating the virtues of enlightened beings rather than worshipping personalities.

Mantras are powerful tools for spiritual development. They connect the disciple with higher realms of consciousness and facilitate the awakening of inner potential.

Benefits of Chanting Mantras

1. **Mental Clarity and Focus**: Regular chanting helps to clear the mind of distractions, promoting mental clarity and focus. It helps in aligning thoughts and creating a peaceful mind.
2. **Stress Reduction**: Chanting mantras can lower stress levels by calming the nervous system and reducing the production of stress hormones.
3. **Emotional Healing:** Mantras can release emotional blockages, leading to emotional stability and healing.
4. **Spiritual Growth**: Chanting connects you to higher states of consciousness and spiritual awareness, fostering a deeper connection with the divine.
5. **Enhanced Concentration**: The repetitive nature of chanting improves concentration and mindfulness, making it easier to stay present in the moment.
6. **Physical Benefits**: Chanting can lower blood pressure, improve heart health, and boost the immune system due to its calming effects on the body.

7. **Vibrational Healing**: The vibrations produced by chanting resonate through the body, promoting healing at a cellular level.

8. **Positive Energy**: Chanting fills the practitioner with positive energy, which can radiate outwards and positively affect the surrounding environment.

9. **Improved Breathing**: The practice of chanting involves deep, rhythmic breathing, which enhances lung capacity and overall respiratory health.

While both affirmations and mantras involve repetition to focus the mind and instil positive energy, their applications and underlying philosophies differ. Affirmations are typically secular and aimed at improving one's mental state and achieving personal goals. They are grounded in modern psychology and self-help methodologies. In contrast, mantras are deeply embedded in spiritual and religious contexts, serving as tools for spiritual awakening, enlightenment, and connection with higher powers.

Affirmations are potent, positive declarations that can revolutionise your mindset, transform your thoughts, and shape your reality. By repeating these empowering statements, one can:

- Rewire the brain to focus on positivity and potential
- Overcome self-doubt, fear and limitations
- Develop an unshakeable confidence and self-belief
- Enhance your resilience, adaptability, and growth mindset
- Attract abundance, success and happiness into your life

Effective affirmations are always:

- Present tense: "I am" instead of "I will be"
- Positive: Focus on what you want, not on what you don't want
- Personal: Use "I" statements to own your truth

- Emotional: Connect with your feelings and desires
- Repeated: Regularly reinforce your affirmations

Examples:

- "I am capable and confident in all I do."
- "I trust myself and my abilities."
- "I am worthy of love, respect and happiness."
- "I am grateful for all the abundance in my life."
- "I am strong and resilient in the face of challenges."

To maximise their impact:

- Speak them aloud with conviction and emotion.
- Repeat them regularly, ideally with visualisation - Focus on a specific area of life or goal.
- Use them in conjunction with other personal growth practices.
- Write them down and display them prominently.

By incorporating affirmations into your daily routine, you can:

- Transform your mindset and empower yourself.
- Unlock your full potential and achieve your goals.

Remember, affirmations are a powerful tool for personal growth and transformation. Use them consistently and watch your life change for the better.

Health Affirmations

1. "I am resilient and radiate vibrant health."
2. "My body effortlessly heals and restores itself."
3. "I fuel my body with nourishing foods and self-love."
4. "My mind and body are in perfect harmony and balance."
5. "I adore my body's unique beauty and strength."

6. "I embrace, celebrate and appreciate my health and wellness journey."
7. "My body is a powerful, self-healing temple, capable of miraculous regeneration!"
8. "I trust my body's infinite wisdom to maintain perfect health and wellness!"

Wealth Affirmations

1. "I am a magnet for abundance, prosperity and limitless wealth!"
2. "My wealth and success skyrocket every day, effortlessly and exponentially!"
3. "I trust my genius-level ability to attract and manage abundance with ease!"
4. "Money flows to me in various ways!"
5. "Money flows to me effortlessly!"
6. "I am the master of my abundance!"

Love affirmations

1. "I am lovable, deserving of unconditional love and respect - always!"
2. "My heart is a boundless, overflowing fountain of love and connection!"
3. "I am in a joyful relationship with everyone around me!"
4. "I attract loving and supportive relationships in my life!"
5. "I am love, loved, and loving!"
6. "I am a source of love and positivity, attracting the same energy into all my relationships!"

My favourite affirmation is:

"I am not busy, I am easy" by BK Shivani:

"I am not busy, I am easy" is a powerful affirmation that shifts your mindset from stress to serenity. Repeating this phrase helps me let go of the need to constantly rush and accomplish. It reminds me that life is not about being busy, but about being present and then effortless. By embracing this affirmation, I began to prioritise ease, calmness, and clarity. I have started to say no to non-essential tasks, and yes to self-care and relaxation. I have made this affirmation a habit, and I am finding my life transforming into a peaceful and joyful journey.

T - TRANSFORMATION

Transformation refers to the deep and lasting changes that occur within an individual as a result of regular meditation practice. This transformation impacts various aspects of a person's life, including their emotional state, cognitive functions, behaviour, spirituality, and physical well-being.

Emotional and Psychological Transformation

Emotional Regulation: Meditation helps individuals manage their emotions by promoting mindfulness and presence. For example, mindfulness meditation encourages observing thoughts and feelings without judgement, which reduces emotional reactivity and builds emotional resilience. Over time, this practice can significantly decrease levels of stress, anxiety and depression.

Enhanced Self-awareness: Practices like Vipassana meditation foster deep self-awareness by helping individuals understand their thought patterns and emotional reactions. This self-awareness is key to personal growth as it enables one to recognise and modify negative behaviours.

Cognitive and Behavioural Transformation

Improved Concentration and Focus: Techniques like focused attention meditation, which involves concentrating on a specific object such as the breath, can sharpen cognitive abilities. Research has shown that regular meditation enhances attention span, memory, and creativity.

Positive Behavioural Changes: Consistent meditation practice often leads to positive behavioural shifts. For example, someone practising loving-kindness meditation (Metta) may become more compassionate and empathetic, leading to kinder and more considerate interactions with others.

Spiritual Transformation

Sense of Oneness: Many meditation practices aim to transcend the ego, leading to a profound sense of unity with the universe. Techniques like transcendental meditation or deep Zen meditation can result in experiences where individuals feel deeply connected to everything around them, fostering inner peace and fulfilment.

Higher States of Consciousness: Advanced meditation can lead to altered states of consciousness, where practitioners may experience profound insights or even enlightenment, perceiving reality beyond ordinary experiences of time and space.

Physical Transformation

Health Benefits: Meditation is associated with numerous physical health benefits, including lower blood pressure, improved immune function, and reduced chronic pain.

These physical changes often complement the mental and emotional benefits, contributing to overall well-being.

Enhanced Body Awareness: Practices like body scan meditation or yoga-based meditation increase body awareness, leading to better posture, reduced physical tension, and improved overall physical health.

Consider someone dealing with chronic stress. Initially, meditation may help them manage their stress responses. With continued practice, they might notice a decrease in their overall anxiety levels, improved reactions to stressful situations, and a general sense of calm and well-being. This transformation can enhance their quality of life, improve relationships, and boost overall health. The transformation that occurs through meditation is a comprehensive process affecting the mind, emotions, behaviour, and body. It requires dedication and an open mind but offers profound, lasting changes that can lead to a more peaceful, aware, and fulfilling life.

I - INTEGRATING

Integration is the process of bringing together diverse elements into a unified whole. Meditation and personal development involve harmonising the mind, body, and spirit to achieve a state of inner peace and balance. Integration requires awareness, acceptance, and the ability to synthesise different aspects of oneself into a cohesive, functioning unity.

True spiritual growth and inner peace can only be achieved through the harmonious integration of the mind, body, and soul. Fragmentation of these elements leads to internal conflict and disharmony, preventing individuals from realising their full potential and experiencing true tranquillity.

Preksha Meditation, for example, fosters this integration. It focuses on the perception of the self through disciplined awareness of one's thoughts, emotions, and bodily sensations. By practising this meditation, individuals learn to observe their internal states without judgement, allowing them to understand and integrate these aspects of themselves more fully.

By the habit of non-violence, truthfulness, and compassion, one can develop a deeper sense of connection within themselves and with the world around them. Ethical living becomes a natural expression of their integrated being, helping them to choose their actions with wisdom.

For instance, integrating ethical principles into daily life can reduce internal conflict and promote a sense of consistency and purpose. This ethical integration, combined with meditative practices, helps individuals achieve a balanced state of being, where the mind is calm, the body is relaxed, and the spirit is uplifted.

In summary, integration is a holistic process that involves harmonising the mind, body, and spirit through meditation, ethical living, and self-awareness. By achieving this integration, individuals can attain inner peace, clarity, and a deeper connection with their true selves, leading to a more enriched and balanced life.

Here is a guided meditation suggested by Acharya Mahapragya that focuses on integration:

Preksha Meditation: A Guided Practice for Integration

1. Preparation:
   - Choose a quiet and comfortable place where you won't be disturbed.
   - Sit in a comfortable position either on a chair or on the floor with your spine straight.
2. Centring Yourself:
   - Close Your Eyes Gently to eliminate external distractions.
   - Begin with a few deep breaths. Inhale deeply through your nose, hold for a moment, and exhale slowly through your mouth. Repeat this a few times to relax your body and mind.
3. Awareness of the Body:
   - Body Scan: Start by bringing your awareness to your toes and gradually move up through your body. Notice any tension or discomfort and consciously relax those areas. Continue this scan until you reach the top of your head.
4. Awareness of the Breath:
   - Breathing Meditation: Focus your attention on your breath. Observe the rhythm of your breathing going in and out without trying to change it. Be fully present with each breath.
5. Concentration on the Centre of Consciousness (Ajna Chakra):
   - Focus on the Forehead: Direct your attention to the centre of your forehead, the Ajna Chakra, also known as the

third eye. This point is believed to be the seat of intuition and higher consciousness.

- Visualization: Visualise a bright, white light spreading and enveloping your entire being, bringing clarity and insight.

6. Mantra Chanting:

- Choose a Mantra that resonates with you. Common mantras include "Aum" or "So Hum."
- Chant Silently: Silently chant the mantra while maintaining your focus on the Ajna Chakra. Let the mantra vibrate through your mind and body, creating a sense of unity and harmony.

7. Integration and Reflection:

- Reflect on Integration: As you meditate, reflect on the concept of integration. Think about how different aspects of your life—mind, body, and spirit—can come together to create a balanced and harmonious existence.
- Embrace Wholeness: Embrace the idea that true peace and inner stillness come from integrating these aspects. Allow this understanding to deepen your meditation practice.

8. Closing the Meditation:

- Slowly bring your awareness back to your surroundings. Feel the weight of your body, feel the chair or the floor where you are sitting.
- Express Gratitude: Take a moment to express gratitude for this time of meditation and the insights you have gained.
- Open Your Eyes: Gently open your eyes and take a few moments to reorient yourself before resuming your daily activities.

Benefits of Preksha Meditation:

- Mental Clarity: Enhances focus and mental clarity by bringing awareness to the present moment.
- Emotional Balance: Helps in managing emotions and reduces stress and anxiety.
- Physical Relaxation: Promotes relaxation and reduces physical tension.
- Spiritual Growth: Deepens the connection with one's inner self and promotes spiritual growth.
- Holistic Integration: Encourages the integration of mind, body, and spirit, leading to a harmonious and peaceful life.

N - NOURISHMENT

Sacred Act of Self-Love

Nourishment refers to the process of providing or receiving sustenance, care, and support for growth, development, and well-being. It encompasses not only physical nutrition but also emotional, mental, and spiritual sustenance. Nourishment involves cultivating a deep sense of self-care, self-love, and connection to oneself, others, and the environment. It is about feeding one's body, mind, and spirit with wholesome experiences, relationships, and activities that promote harmony, balance, and vitality. Through nourishment, we replenish our energies, rejuvenate our spirit, and flourish in all aspects of life, leading to a more fulfilling and purposeful existence.

Let us treat our bodies as sacred temples, nourishing them not just with food, but with the power of mindful breathing, the warmth of a genuine smile, and the deep rest offered by Yoga Nidra.

MINDFUL BREATHING

BREATHING TECHNIQUE - There are several techniques of breathing, such as deep breathing and alternate breathing. These techniques are known to calm the mind and promote relaxation. When these techniques are practiced mindfully, and we understand the effects of inhaling, exhaling, and holding our breath, we gain better control over our breathing. Let's delve into the aspects of breathing and how pranayama nourishes our body.

Understanding Breathing Phases

1. **Inhalation (Puraka)**: During inhalation, oxygen is drawn into the lungs, where it is absorbed into the bloodstream.

This process energises the body and mind, preparing them for action.

2. **Exhalation (Rechaka)**: Exhaling releases carbon dioxide and other waste gases from the body. This process helps to cleanse the system and promotes relaxation.

3. **Breath Retention (Kumbhaka)**: Holding the breath, either after inhalation or exhalation, can increase lung capacity and improve oxygen exchange in the lungs. This practice also helps to develop control over the breath and can enhance concentration and focus.

Pranayama: Nourishing the Body Pranayama, the practice of breath control in yoga, is a powerful tool for nourishing the body. By regulating the breath, pranayama techniques can enhance the flow of prana (life force) throughout the body, promoting physical and mental health. Pranayama can improve respiratory function, boost immune response, and reduce stress and anxiety.

By incorporating deep breathing and alternate nostril breathing into our daily routine, we can achieve a balanced state of mind and body. Understanding and practising these breathing techniques helps us gain better control over our breath, promoting overall well-being and inner peace.

Deep Breathing Deep breathing involves taking slow, deep breaths, filling the lungs, and then exhaling slowly. This technique increases oxygen intake, calms the nervous system, and helps reduce stress. Practising deep breathing regularly can improve lung capacity, enhance mental clarity, and promote overall well-being.

Alternate Nostril Breathing Alternate nostril breathing, or Nadi Shodhana, involves inhaling through one nostril while closing the other and then switching. This technique balances the right and left hemispheres of the brain, promoting mental clarity and emotional stability. It also helps to calm the mind, reduce anxiety, and improve concentration.

SMILE

A smile is a simple yet profound facial expression that conveys warmth, happiness, and friendliness. When the corners of your mouth curve upward, it's a universal sign of goodwill that transcends language barriers. Smiles can express a variety of emotions, from joy and amusement to gratitude and affection. As a fundamental form of non-verbal communication, smiling helps build connections and fosters social bonds.

The Transformation Through My Smile: A Personal Journey

Embracing My Smile and Its Impact on My Life

Growing up, I was self-conscious about my smile. My big teeth and visible gums made me hesitant to fully express myself, especially during my teenage years. I often found myself holding back, not wanting to draw attention to what I saw as a flaw. This insecurity led to a lack of confidence, and I started to withdraw socially. My reluctance to smile freely made others perceive me as shy and introverted, further reinforcing my self-doubt.

However, my family always saw my smile differently. They praised my white teeth and told me that my natural smile was a gift, even joking that I could be the face of a toothpaste ad. Yet, it wasn't until my husband entered my life that I began to see my smile in a new light. He adored my smile, calling it infectious and saying it brightened his day. His constant encouragement helped me embrace my smile, and with that, I began to notice profound changes within myself.

How My Smile Nourished Me

As I started to smile more confidently, I noticed subtle yet powerful changes in my body and mind:

- **Increased Confidence**: The more I smiled, the more I began to believe in my worth. Smiling made me feel empowered, shifting my focus from my insecurities to my strengths. I realised that my smile wasn't just a physical expression—it was a reflection of my inner joy and confidence.
- **Reduced Stress**: Smiling became a natural stress reliever. In moments of anxiety or self-doubt, smiling helped me calm down and regain control. The simple act of smiling triggered a sense of relaxation, allowing me to face challenges with a clearer mind and a lighter heart.
- **Enhanced Positivity**: With each smile, I felt a surge of positivity. My outlook on life became more optimistic, and I started to attract positive experiences and relationships. Smiling shifted my mindset from one of fear and doubt to one of hope and possibility.
- **Strengthened Connections**: As I smiled more openly, I noticed that others responded to me differently. My smile became a bridge, helping me connect with people on a deeper level. I went from feeling isolated to being surrounded by a community of friends who appreciated my warmth and authenticity.
- **Physical Well-being**: Smiling not only improved my emotional state but also had a tangible impact on my physical health. I felt more energised, and my overall well-being improved. The tension I once carried in my body began to melt away, replaced by a sense of ease and contentment.

Ripple Effect of My Smile

The transformation didn't stop with me. As I embraced my smile, I began to share it with others. My husband's words about my smile being infectious became a reality—I noticed how my smile could lift someone's spirits, spark a conversation, or even brighten a stranger's day. The positivity I felt inside radiated outward, creating a ripple effect of joy and connection.

In the end, what started as a source of insecurity became my greatest asset. My smile nourished me, helping me grow into a more confident, positive, and connected person. I am grateful to my parents and husband for helping me see the beauty in my smile and for encouraging me to embrace it fully. Today, I smile not just for myself but for the joy it brings to others. My smile is a reflection of the inner peace and happiness I have found, and I am committed to sharing that with the world.

By understanding the profound impact that smiling can have on our lives, we can all learn to embrace and nurture our unique smiles, allowing them to transform us from the inside out.

SIX Smile Prescription Programme:

1. Recognise and acknowledge your current smile habits. You can practice by smiling in front of the mirror for 30 seconds every day and then observing how you feel. Walk with a smile and observe how others respond.
2. Practice exercises to stimulate smiling, such as watching comedies or reading funny stories.
3. Gratitude is the biggest source of strength to smile. Cultivate a habit of writing at least three things you are grateful for with a smile as you think about them.
4. The Smile and Breathe Exercise: Inhale deeply, smile, and exhale slowly, repeating the process.
5. The Fake-It-Till-You-Make-It: Force a smile, even when you don't feel like it, to trick your brain into feeling happier.
6. Spread positivity by sharing your smile with others.

SLEEP

Sleep is a natural state where your mind and body rest. As you fall asleep, your mind disconnects from your senses

and muscles, gradually leading to a loss of awareness of the outside world.

Consistency in sleep is like building a strong foundation for your day, just as lizards follow their natural rhythms.

Going to bed and waking up at the same time each day gives your body a reliable schedule, much like how lizards stick to their internal clock rhythms that respond to light and darkness, highlighting the significance of maintaining a natural sleep-wake cycle.

There's a difference between waking up refreshed and energised versus feeling groggy and tired.

Quality sleep isn't just about the hours logged – it's about how rejuvenating those hours are. Lizards teach us to conserve energy by resting during the hottest parts of the day, reminding us that strategic rest is vital. When you prioritise sleep, it's like the ultimate life hack, turning you into a beacon of focus and tranquillity. Imagine waking up with your mind as clear as a sunny day, effortlessly breezing through tasks with razor-sharp concentration. Just like lizards adapt to their environment, your body and mind benefit from a calm and consistent sleep routine.

Sleep is also your emotional anchor, helping you stay centred and balanced. Lizards instinctively know when to hibernate, illustrating the importance of taking breaks during tough times. This translates to us allowing our minds and bodies the rest they need to maintain emotional stability and reduce stress, creating the perfect environment for meditation.

In the same way, lizards choose simple, sheltered spots for sleep, you should aim for a clutter-free sleep environment. A well-rested body is like a well-maintained vehicle, ready to handle the challenges of the day without any issues. When you wake up feeling positive and energised, it's a sign that your sleep is doing its job—just like how a lizard's simple but effective sleep habits keep it ready for the day ahead.

With sufficient sleep, your brain goes into overdrive, excelling in everything from memory recall to problem-solving. It's as if sleep gives you a mental upgrade, making meditation techniques and daily tasks feel like a breeze. Physically, sleep works wonders too, relaxing your muscles so you can sit comfortably during meditation without discomfort.

Even your hormones are kept in perfect balance, thanks to a good night's rest. This means stress levels stay low, providing the mental stability needed for successful meditation sessions. Plus, a well-rested body is a healthy body, keeping you on track with your meditation practice without any interruptions.

Good sleep sets the stage for a day filled with clarity, calm, and positivity, making meditation not just possible but genuinely enjoyable.

Ultimately, the best indicator of good sleep is how you feel the next day. If you find yourself cheerfully humming along to your morning playlist rather than reaching for that third cup of coffee before 10 a.m., you've nailed it. Good sleep isn't just restful—it's downright rejuvenating, setting the stage for a day that's a little brighter, a little sharper, and a whole lot more productive.

YOGA NIDRA

Yoga Nidra is a structured technique designed to bring about deep physical, mental, and emotional relaxation. Often referred to as "psychic sleep" or "conscious sleep," it allows you to remain awake while reaching a deeply restful state, connecting with your subconscious and unconscious mind. In this practice, the mind becomes more open and receptive.

Just like molten iron can be moulded into a desired shape, during Yoga Nidra, the mind enters a state where it becomes flexible, allowing you to instil positive and creative impressions. This is possible because the mind's usual distractions and mental chatter are quieted, making it highly sensitive to suggestions.

Yoga Nidra awakens the emotional layers of the mind, allowing for deeper transformation and relaxation.

By tapping into this relaxed, open state, one can access insights and intuitive knowledge that might not be available during regular consciousness. This unique quality of Yoga Nidra enhances self-awareness and helps to reset mental patterns.

Yoga Nidra offers a wide range of benefits, making it both powerful and surprisingly enjoyable. One of its key advantages is deep relaxation, helping you to recharge in a way that regular sleep can't. For instance, imagine feeling completely refreshed after just 20 minutes of Yoga Nidra—like a power nap, but with more lasting calm.

It also helps reduce stress by calming your nervous system. For example, someone with high anxiety might feel like they've hit a mental reset button after a session. Another benefit is mental clarity. If you're juggling multiple thoughts at once, Yoga Nidra can clear the mental clutter and allow you to focus better.

Before each chemotherapy session, Vikram's mind would race with endless anxious thoughts, causing a lot of stress. However, when he began practising Yoga Nidra, things took a profound turn. Just as a lizard remains still and calm, fully in the present moment while observing its surroundings, Vikram found the ability to quiet his anxious mind through Yoga Nidra, creating a peaceful environment despite the challenges he faced. After each session, he would awaken with a calm and stable mind. It not only helped him relax physically but also shifted his mental state, making the entire environment more peaceful and supportive for both of us, which had a positive impact on both our emotional well-being during those challenging times.

G - GROUNDING

Grounding is the process of connecting oneself to the present moment and the physical world, fostering stability and balance. It involves techniques that help anchor the mind and body, allowing one to feel secure, centred, and in harmony with the environment.

Grounding helps individuals stay present and reduces feelings of anxiety or disorientation. For example, after a stressful day, one might feel overwhelmed and disconnected. Practising grounding techniques, such as standing barefoot on the earth, can help realign the body's energy, providing a sense of stability and calm.

As I embarked on my grounding journey, I was filled with curiosity and a hint of scepticism. But, with each passing day, I began to experience the profound benefits of reconnecting with the Earth's natural energy.

Vikram's hesitancy and fear of getting an infection due to grounding was a turning point for me. Many people had suggested that he practice grounding, but unfortunately, he didn't take action immediately. His experience taught me the importance of taking action and being proactive about my well-being.

It was Mr Yunus Shipchandler and his wife Dr Durriya, founders of The Hidden Oasis, Pune, who facilitated the Freedom from Diabetes residential retreat at their resort, introduced me to the concept of grounding. They shared their knowledge and expertise, and I'm forever grateful for their guidance.

Grounding, also known as Earthing, is a holistic practice that involves making direct contact with the Earth's surface to promote physical, mental, and emotional well-being. By doing so, we can:

Reduce stress and anxiety, calming our nervous system and promoting relaxation.

Improve sleep quality by regulating our sleep patterns and waking up feeling refreshed

Relieve pain, reduce inflammation, and alleviate chronic pain

NO INFLAMMATION + DEEP SLEEP = NO DISEASES

Boost our immune system, neutralising free radicals and promoting overall well-being

Increase energy, reduce fatigue, and enhance vitality

Support cardiovascular health, lower blood pressure, and improve blood flow

Enhance our mood, reducing symptoms of depression and anxiety.

Increase our sense of calm and well-being, promoting feelings of relaxation and connection to nature.

As I began to practise grounding, I felt a sense of trepidation, but with each passing day, I grew more confident. I started with short sessions, gradually increasing the duration as I became more comfortable. I combined grounding with deep breathing, meditation, and yoga, and soon it became an integral part of my self-care routine.

If you're curious about grounding, I encourage you to take the first step. Find a safe location, take off your shoes, and connect with the Earth's natural energy. You might be surprised at the profound benefits you experience.

Ways to Practice Grounding:

- Walk barefoot outdoors.
- Sit or lie on the ground,
- Use a grounding mat or sheet indoors.
- Swim in a lake or ocean.
- Practice yoga or meditation outdoors.

- Take a warm bath with Epsom salts.
- Wear grounding shoes or accessories.

I'd like to extend my heartfelt gratitude to Mr. Yunus and Dr. Durriya for introducing me to the concept of grounding. Their guidance and expertise have been invaluable, and I'm grateful for their contribution to my well-being journey.

CHAPTER 6

PRACTICES

Before entering practice, there are some general suggestions that we need to follow before starting the meditation process or peaceful practice.

1. The room should be properly ventilated. If a fan or air conditioner is required, make sure you are not in direct contact, especially if practices are for longer periods, particularly in yoga Nidra because body temperature tends to reduce during the relaxation process.
2. If practices are done at the same time, it can harness the power of neuroplasticity to rewire and regulate neurotransmitters like dopamine and serotonin. This leads to training our mind to enter into specific frequencies of alpha, beta, theta, delta promoting relaxation, focus, or deep sleep.
3. If you are a beginner, regular lessons should be taken by qualified teachers. A teacher knows what kind of practice will suit a particular student. For example, if a student is tense, then a relaxation technique will be applied, but if the student is already relaxed, then deep meditation practice will be conducted.
4. The best time to practice is early morning or before going to bed (to have a refreshing sleep).

5. Meditation like yoga Nidra should be practiced on an empty stomach or after three hours of heavy meals and half an hour after light refreshment because in this practice, the body temperature drops very fast, leading to a reduction in digestive enzymes. A reduction in digestive enzymes can lead to impaired nutrient absorption and digestive disorders like bloating, gas, abdominal pain, and fatigue.

Anything in life can fail you, but not the intention made during relaxation. Everyone has many dreams, ambitions, and desires. However, most of them get lost, exhausted, and destroyed, just as when you scatter seeds in different places. Some may grow, but most will die. Intention is a seed that you create and then sow in your mind.

PRACTICE NO. 1

Composed Breathing

1. Focus on the breath: Bring your attention to your breath, feeling the sensation of the air entering and leaving your nostrils.
2. Let go of thoughts: When your mind wanders, gently acknowledge the thought and let it go, returning your focus to the breath.
3. Be present in the body: Feel the breath moving in and out of your body, observing any physical sensations without judgement.
4. Use the breath as an anchor: When your mind wanders, use the breath as an anchor to bring your attention back to the present moment.
5. Don't control the breath: Allow your breath to happen naturally; allow things to be as they are without trying to change them.

6. Feel the breath moving in and out of your body and observe physical sensations

6. Focus on the present moment: Don't identify with your thoughts, emotions, or physical sensations - simply observe them.

7. Let go of past regrets or future worries and simply be present in the moment with your breath.

By practising this technique, you can cultivate a deeper sense of presence, calmness, and inner peace. Remember, the goal is not to achieve a specific state, but to simply be present in the moment.

PRACTICE NO. 2

Chanting Of Any Mantra

- Find a Quiet Space: Sit comfortably in a quiet room.
- Set an Intention: Focus on inner peace and calmness.
- Posture and Breath: Sit with a straight spine, eyes closed, and take deep breaths.
- Focus on the Mantra: Chant slowly and feel the vibration.

Use a mala for chanting a mantra. Begin by holding the mala, typically made of 108 beads, and locate the off-bead known as the meru. Bring the tips of your ring finger and thumb together, letting the mala rest at this point, with your palm resting on your knee. As you chant your chosen mantra, such as "Om," use your middle finger and thumb to turn each bead toward yourself, leaving the index finger apart, as it represents duality. When you complete 108 repetitions and return to the meru bead, avoid crossing it. Instead, turn the mala around and continue by starting the next cycle from the bead you ended on, completing another round of japa.

- Consistency: Continue chanting for 10 minutes.
- End with Gratitude: Sit in silence for a moment, feeling the effects of the chant, and express gratitude for the practice.

PRACTICE NO.3

Writing a gratitude journal entry:

1. Choose a quiet and comfortable space to sit and reflect.
2. Date your entry to track your progress and reflect on past experiences.
3. Write down 3-5 things you're grateful for, no matter how small they may seem. Be specific and detailed.
4. Explain why you're grateful for each item. How did it positively impact your life?
5. Elaborate on the emotions you feel when thinking about each blessing.
6. Reflect on how your life would be different without these blessings.
7. End with a positive affirmation or a message of gratitude to yourself or others.
8. Close your entry with a thoughtful phrase or a simple "Thank you."
9. Take a moment to review your entry, feeling the emotions and absorbing the positivity.
10. Keep your journal private and make it a sacred space for your thoughts and feelings.

Remember, consistency is key! Aim to write in your gratitude journal at the same time every day to make it a habit.

PRACTICE NO.4

Guided affirmations with positive words used during both inhalation and exhalation:

Health affirmations

Inhale: "I am worthy of vibrant health"

Exhale: "I release all limitations, embracing perfect wellness."

REPEAT: "I am healthy, I am energised, I am radiant, I am well-nourished, I am strong."

"I trust my body's infinite wisdom to maintain perfect health and wellness!"

Wealth affirmations

Inhale: "I am worthy of abundance"

Exhale: "I release all scarcity, embracing prosperity."

Repeat: "I am a wealth magnet, I am a success powerhouse, I am unstoppable!"

"I trust that I will attract soulmate relationships that uplift and inspire me!"

Love affirmations

Inhale: "I am worthy of love"

Exhale: "I release all fear, embracing unconditional love."

Repeat: "I am lovable, I am worthy of love, I am a magnet for soulmate connections!"

By using positive words during exhalation, you're reinforcing the release of limitations and embracing the desired outcome. This amplifies the effectiveness of the affirmations and helps to rewire your mind with empowering beliefs.

CREATE YOUR PERSONALISED AFFIRMATION

Develop statements that resonate with your personal experiences and aspirations. Ensure they are positive, specific, and stated in the present tense.

Use your experiences to craft affirmations that reflect your journey and the growth you've achieved.

Dedicate specific times each day for your affirmation practice, such as morning routines, before bed, or during moments of reflection.

Creating a consistent habit helps reinforce the positive messages.

Example:

"Just as I overcame my insecurities about my smile, I can overcome any challenge with confidence and grace."

For this, I would stand in front of the mirror, look into my eyes, and say my affirmations out loud.

- "My unique smile is a beautiful expression of my true self."
- "I am confident and proud of who I am, and my smile reflects my inner strength."
- "Each day, I embrace my smile more fully, and it brings joy to myself and those around me."
- "I am thankful for the support of my family and loved ones who help me shine my brightest smile."

By integrating these practices into my daily life, I could harness the power of affirmations to continue nurturing my self-confidence, embracing my unique smile, and spreading positivity to those around me. Affirmations, combined with an authentic smile, can lead to a more fulfilling and joyful existence.

PRACTICE NO. 5

The **Yoga Nidra** technique by **Swami Satyananda Saraswati** is a deep relaxation and meditation practice. For beginners, the script typically follows a guided process where you gradually move into a state of complete relaxation, maintaining awareness as you transition from wakefulness to deep rest.

1. **Introduction & Preparation:**
   - Lie down in **Shavasana** (corpse pose), on your back, arms slightly away from the body, palms facing up.
   - Settle comfortably and close your eyes.
   - Focus on stillness and relax the entire body.
2. **Sankalpa (Resolve):**
   - A short positive statement or intention (Sankalpa) is mentally repeated three times. For beginners, this could be as simple as "I am peaceful" or "I am calm."
3. **Body Scan (Rotation of Consciousness):**
   - The instructor will guide you through a rotation of awareness through different parts of the body. You mentally focus on each part as mentioned, starting from the right side of the body (right thumb, fingers, arm, etc.), and moving across to the left side, head, and down to the feet.
4. **Breath Awareness:**
   - Bring awareness to your natural breath. Simply observe the breath without changing it. For beginners, this practice cultivates calmness and focus.
   - Sometimes, awareness is focused on counting breaths, particularly in areas like the abdomen, chest, or nostrils.

5. **Opposites (Pairs of Opposites):**

   - You are guided to experience contrasting sensations like heaviness and lightness, heat and cold, etc. This enhances your awareness of the body and mind.

6. **Visualizations:**

   - The instructor guides visualizations to deepen mental relaxation. Beginners might visualise simple objects or calming scenes, such as a serene lake, open sky, or a candle flame.

7. **Sankalpa (Resolve) – Repeated:**

   - At the end of the practice, the Sankalpa is repeated again, allowing it to settle into the subconscious mind.

8. **Ending the Practice:**

   - Gradually bring awareness back to the body and surroundings. Wiggle your fingers and toes, stretch gently, and slowly open your eyes when ready.

Duration: The practice typically lasts 20-30 minutes for beginners.

PRACTICE NO. 6

BETTER SLEEP PRACTICES

Improving sleep quality is like setting the stage for a nightly performance where your body and mind can fully relax and rejuvenate. Here are some techniques that make the process not only effective but also enjoyable:

1. **Body Scan**: Imagine lying down and mentally scanning your body like a soothing spotlight moving from head to toe. As you focus on each body part, let go of any tension, as if you're deflating a balloon. Start with your toes and slowly work your way up to your head, feeling the relaxation spread like a warm wave.

2. **Yoga Nidra**: Picture yourself sinking into a cosy hammock of relaxation. Yoga Nidra, or yogic sleep, is like having a personal guide lead you through a journey of deep rest. It's a bit like a guided meditation but for sleep, where you effortlessly drift into a state of profound calm, leaving your mind and body fully refreshed.
3. **Avoid Stimulating Activities**: Think of your pre-bedtime routine as a gentle wind-down rather than a time for high-energy activities. Swap out scrolling through your phone or engaging in intense debates for something more calming, like reading a light book or listening to soft music. It's like preparing your mind for sleep by dimming the lights on your day.
4. **Create a Sleep-Conducive Environment**: Turn your bedroom into the ultimate sleep sanctuary. Think of it as designing a cosy retreat—dim the lights, keep the room cool, and banish noise. It's like crafting the perfect setting for a night of uninterrupted, blissful sleep.
5. **Consistent Sleep Schedule**: Establish a sleep routine like a well-oiled machine. Going to bed and waking up at the same time every day, even on weekends, is like training your body's internal clock to work in your favour. Over time, you'll find yourself naturally drifting off and waking up with ease, no alarm necessary.
6. **Inner Engineering**: Picture yourself fine-tuning your inner energies like a well-maintained engine. Through practices like meditation and yoga, you can balance these energies, making sleep a natural and effortless process. It's like tuning an instrument—when everything is in harmony, sleep comes naturally.
7. **Reverse Counting**: Counting sheep might be old-school, but reverse counting is the new trick. Start at 100 and count backward to 1, like unravelling a mental thread. If you lose

track, no worries—just start again. It's a simple yet effective way to quiet the mind and drift off.

By incorporating these techniques into your nightly routine, along with a balanced lifestyle filled with a healthy diet, regular exercise, and stress management, you'll set yourself up for consistently good sleep. It's like having all the ingredients for a perfect night's rest, leading to brighter, more energetic days ahead.

PRACTICE NO. 7

A GROUNDING YOGA POSE (TREE POSE)

Grounding is closely linked to the Root Chakra (Muladhara), located at the base of the spine. This chakra is responsible for feelings of safety, security, and connection to the earth. When balanced, it promotes stability and a sense of being grounded.

Tree Pose (Vrikshasana)

- Chakra Involvement: The Root Chakra is activated in this pose as it emphasises stability and grounding through the feet.
- Mudra Connection: Gyan Mudra, where the tip of the index finger touches the thumb while other fingers remain straight, can be used. This mudra, when practiced in standing poses, enhances grounding and focus.

Imagine feeling anxious before a big presentation. To ground yourself, you might:

1. Stand Barefoot: Remove your shoes and stand barefoot on the ground.
2. Visualise Roots: Close your eyes and visualize roots extending from your feet deep into the Earth.
3. Gyan Mudra: Form the Gyan Mudra with your hands to enhance focus and grounding.

4. Deep Breaths: Take slow, deep breaths, inhaling through your nose and exhaling through your mouth, calming your mind and body.
5. Affirmation: Repeat a grounding affirmation, such as "I am safe, secure, and connected to the earth."

By incorporating this grounding technique, one can achieve a state of calmness, balance, and present-moment awareness, essential for effective meditation and overall well-being.

CONCLUSION

As we journey through life's twists and turns, may we remember the power of peaceful presence. May we cultivate gratitude, affirmation, intention, visualization, and mindfulness to guide us on our path.

Here is a poem that captures the essence of our journey.

NAVIGATING PEACEFUL PRESENCE

In life's vast ocean, we sail and roam

with a peaceful presence, our heart finds home.

A gentle compass, guiding us through,

Calm and clear, in all we do

With grateful hearts, we embrace each day

and affirm our worth in every way.

We set our intentions, pure and bright

and visualise our dreams, taking flight

with mindful breaths, we ride the tide

and find stillness, where love resides.

In the darkest night, we navigate with ease

And find the stars in peaceful seas.

May these words inspire you to continue navigating life's challenges with a peaceful presence. Remember, peace is always within you, guiding your home.

www.ingramcontent.com/pod-product-compliance
Lightning Source LLC
LaVergne TN
LVHW091033150826
845672LV00006BA/1796

* 9 7 9 8 8 9 6 3 2 4 5 5 3 *